LUEDER JACHENS, MD, born in Bremen in 1951, p.... anthroposophical medical student groups whilst studying medicine in Goettingen and Kiel. He specialized in dermatology and allergology, then worked in medical departments at an anthroposophical hospital. He has worked in private practice as a skin specialist in Stiefenhofen/ Allgaeu, Germany since 1992, and developed the Christophorus Medical Centre.

Healing the Skin

Holistic approaches to treating skin conditions

A practical guide based on anthroposophic medicine

Lueder Jachens

Translated and edited by Anna R. Meuss, FCIL

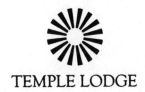

TEMPLE LODGE

Temple Lodge Publishing
Hillside House, The Square
Forest Row, RH18 5ES

www.templelodge.com

Published by Temple Lodge 2008

Originally published in German under the title *Hautkrankheiten ganzheitlich heilen* by Verlag Freies Geistesleben, Stuttgart. This translation is based on the second revised edition, 2006

A catalogue record for this book is available from the British Library

ISBN 978 1902636 91 7

Cover by Andrew Morgan Design
Typeset by DP Photosetting, Neath, West Glamorgan
Printed and bound by Cromwell Press Ltd., Trowbridge, Wiltshire

CONTENTS

CONTENTS

CONTENTS

IMPORTANT NOTE

This book cannot take the place of a skin specialist.

All treatments that require medical supervision are therefore labelled (P) for physician.

The symbol (S) for self-medication stands for measures patients can take for themselves without consulting a physician.

Superscript figures refer to products of the following manufacturers:

[1] Weleda

[2] Wala

All the information given in this book has been carefully checked and is in accord with the latest established knowledge. Recommendations of medicines or treatments are based on subjective choice, with no claim for completeness. They reflect the author's practice as a dermatologist. Trade or registered names are mentioned claiming the freedom of the press and without regard to manufacturers' interests; there is no intention to advertise them.

Details on medicines and treatment measures are given with the proviso that dosages and methods of use may change in time as new knowledge is gained in research, with clinical experience and changes in the availability of products. Freedom from human error or errata can never be claimed, and liability can therefore not be accepted for details concerning use or dosages, nor for the actions of the products. It is most important always to check the details given in this book against manufacturers' information on leaflets enclosed with their products and take note of recommended doses and contraindications as stated by the manufacturers. The author and the publishers take no legal responsibility for damage to persons or property.

It should also be noted that a physician should always be consulted in case of doubt, especially if symptoms persist for several days. The information given in this book is neither designed nor suitable to take the place of such a consultation.

TRANSLATOR'S NOTE

This book is an *edited* translation of the German original, as medical and other care provisions differ between countries. This has resulted in some minor omissions and some added information (marked Tr. for translator).

Weleda, Wala, Dr Hauschka and Birkencreme sources in several countries have been consulted to check on the names and availability of their products in English-speaking countries. I am especially indebted to the author, who helped me to find contacts, and to Judith Klahre-Parker, PhD, from Weleda (UK) Ltd, who has painstakingly gone through my long lists of products to check for names and availability. I'd also like to thank my colleague Margot Saar who has carefully checked the manuscript for those little errors that will escape attention unless a second pair of eyes is there to spot them, and made some helpful suggestions.

Anna R. Meuss

Contemplating nature
always heed both one and all—
nothing is inside, nothing outside;
for the inside is also outside.
Thus without delay uncover
the sacred open secret.

Johann Wolfgang von Goethe

INTRODUCTION

Seeing the skin in a new way from the anthroposophical point of view

Some very good publications are available to advise lay people today, showing the dermatological and cosmetic means available to deal with skin conditions. The good reason for adding yet another book is that new possibilities arise when natural-scientific medicine is complemented by the insights gained through anthroposophy. This widens our horizons and shows up relationships between the skin and the organism as a whole, and also between skin and psyche, in a way that is not possible if we limit ourselves to the natural-scientific approach.

The first part of this book offers a description of the image that the skin presents from the anthroposophical point of view. In the second part, the most common skin conditions are considered as well as existing possibilities of treating them with the methods of anthroposophical medicine.

At the beginning of the new millennium, people are exposed to an infinite variety of stresses at different levels of their existence. Chemically synthesized substances—some 'identical' with the natural substance, though definitely not to be found in nature—need to be coped with in metabolism at the physical level. Daily life is hectic and lacking in rhythm, which saps people's vitality. A flood of stimuli and innumerable short-lived human contact situations have to be dealt with in the psyche. At the spiritual level of existence, people feel the need to live their own biography, be independent and individual, and no longer socially embedded in a village, town, occupational group, and so on, as was the case just a hundred years ago. Today's environment presents us with all of the above, and to digest them we need to be sound in mind, soul and body.

We are also more than ever challenged to set boundaries for ourselves in both soul and body, with 'boundary problems' arising when we fail to do so. Such a problem may 'turn inwards', affecting the stomach, for instance, with too much acid, or indeed actual gastritis.

1

Or it may affect the skin, causing an eruption. Here we have the deeper causes of the increase in allergies and many different skin conditions.

We may truly speak of skin diseases of our time, for the growing incidence is due to the life we lead today, above all where neuro-dermatitis and melanoma are concerned.

Many people therefore feel that they have good reason to get as much information as possible about the skin and the issues connected with skin diseases. The aim of this book is to meet that wish, providing information from the point of view and the experience of a skin specialist who knows from daily practice the great help, encourage-ment and challenges which the anthroposophical view of the human being offers by putting medicine on a broader basis.

On the other hand, this book cannot replace the skin specialist. Measures that need to be initiated by a physician are therefore clearly labelled (P), for physician. The symbol (S) stands for self-medication, that is, measures patients can use on their own, without first consulting a physician or specialist.

Health care provision has gone through major changes in the six years since the first edition of the book appeared. Many of the therapies used in the holistic approach to medicine are no longer reimbursed by health insurance companies, and that also applies to almost all medi-cines used in anthroposophical medicine. This means an additional burden for people who decide on anthroposophical medical treatment. Politicians have ignored the principle of pluralism for the scientific approaches to medicine.

These developments have evidently been unrealistic and unfair, yet they also have their good side. They encourage people to take responsibility for their own health. Your physical body is a 'temple of God', the instrument that the soul uses in this life to achieve the tasks it has set for itself in the present biography. It needs personal initiative to care for it. The aim of this book is to support such personal initiative, a power which arises directly from the I, the self, of modern human beings. The very act of taking such an initiative already has a powerful healing and health-giving effect.

My thanks go to Drs Franziska Roemer, Hans Werner, Dieter Krahl and Peter Ries for their critical review of the first edition and many important suggestions. I am indebted to Dr Christoph M. Schempp for suggestions relating to the external use of St John's wort, Dr Ulrich Meyer for information on anthroposophical pharmacy.

This book is dedicated to my wife, family physician Christa-Johanna Bub-Jachens, MD, who died in 2003. We had many fruitful talks in the twelve years we worked intensively together in Stiefenhofen Group Practice, and these contributed much to the foundations for this book.

Lueder Jachens
Stiefenhofen, Allgaeu
Spring 2006

Reminder of markers

(S)　For self-medication, without first consulting a physician or specialist.

(P)　Consult a physician or specialist.

[1]　　Weleda product

[2]　　Wala product

['Tr.' indicates information for the English-speaking world added by the translator.]

The seat of the soul
is where inner and outer world touch.
It is at every point
where the two interact.
                                    Novalis

THE HUMAN SKIN

Today, one cannot refer to the physical, material aspect of man and nature without also considering the extensive findings of modern science. The cultural development of humanity is inevitably moving towards developing a highly differentiated scientific method for the study of man and nature based on perceptions made via the human sense organs.

The method used in natural science is that of analysis, where a whole is divided and broken up into its parts. If we apply this to the human skin we gain dermatological (skin specialist) knowledge based mainly on histology (study of body tissues) under the microscope, and at a more subtle level on biochemistry, which is the study of vital processes in a living organ using chemical methods. We will begin by presenting the reader with the knowledge gained in this way.

We will then consider the image of the human skin that arises when medical knowledge is broadened through anthroposophy.

Anatomy of the skin

Three layers are usually distinguished—the epidermis with its horn (keratinized) cells, the elastic dermis or corium which can cope with mechanical stresses, and the subcutis which stores fat and provides padding and warmth.

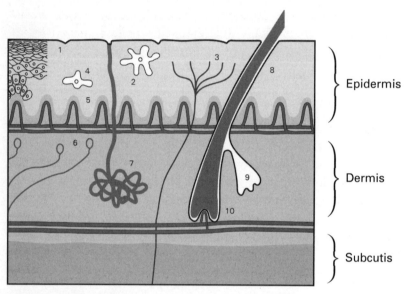

Structure of the skin
1 Horn cells | 2 Defence cell | 3 Nerve fibres | 4 Pigment-producing cell | 5 Papillae with blood vessels | 6 Sensory cells | 7 Sweat glands | 8 Hair | 9 Sebaceous gland | 10 Hair follicle (root)

The epidermis

Under the microscope we see that the epidermis consists of two zones. In a basal layer, epithelial cells sitting side by side like paving stones are continually dividing and simply full of vitality. They obtain the substances they need for their metabolism from the nutrient stream which comes close to the epidermis in the fine capillaries of the upper corium or dermis. Epidermis and dermis are merely separated by a thin basal membrane.

Continuous cell division produces new cells all the time, and as they mature these are pushed up through the layers of the epidermis until they reach the surface. They produce a hornlike, cornified substance, a protein, for the inside of the cell and give off fat lamellae to the outside, into the space between cells. Vitality is gradually lost in the process, as can be seen from the fact that cell nuclei get smaller and smaller and finally break down. In the uppermost layer, the zona cornea, the horn cells are shed as dead squames, or flaky skin scales.

Normal skin will therefore always shed fine flakes which are consistently the same, and our daily environment is full of these. They make up a large proportion of house dust and are eaten by house mites. Ten grams of dander are produced daily by the skin, which is two thousand million horn cells a day. The maturing of substances and death of horn cells thus happen at the same time in the epidermis.

Under normal conditions it is 28 days, a moon cycle, from the birth of a new horn cell in the basal layer to it being shed on the surface. The moon influences all vital and growth processes in the natural world, and its effect is modified every few days as it passes through the zodiac. The vitality of the epidermis and its hair therefore also bears the signature of the moon.

This rhythm is not, of course, governed from outside by the moon we see in the sky at night. It is based on the laws governing the moon; the human organism has made these its own, incorporating them into

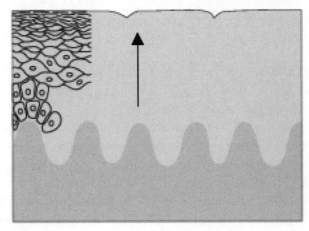

Migration of horn cells through the epidermis

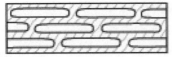

Horn cells and fat lamellae

its time body. It is therefore our inner moon which sets the 28-day rhythm.

In the middle zones of the epidermis, horn cells develop a hexagonal form (seen from above). We see the same hexagonal form in honeycombs and rock crystal; an inner relationship shows itself between processes in the epidermis and in beehives and quartz. These processes have to do with light and warmth.

Horn and fat must mature properly in the epidermis if the skin is to protect us from foreign substances and prevent the body's own substances leaking out. Lack of some biochemical compounds in the fat lamellae between horn cells may mean that the skin is more easily attacked and damaged by the weather, by soap, etc.

Water is chemically bound between the cells in the horny layer of the epidermis (about 10–20% of the matter making up the layer is water). It is bound mainly by urea, a product of protein metabolism; metabolism is highly active wherever sufficient urea is present. The skin's variable ability to hold water serves as an indicator for its vitality. For vital processes always depend on water. If the horny layer is depleted of urea, for instance in someone with a constitutional tendency to develop neurodermatitis, the skin dries up; water is lost to the outside.

Other kinds of cells are also found in the epidermis. Nerve fibres run between the horn cells, their free nerve endings penetrating to its middle layers. This means that the nervous system extends to within fractions of millimetres of the skin surface. A finger stroking the skin is practically touching those sensitive nerves and it is sensed by them. There are 150 free nerve endings to every square centimetre of skin. The combined length of nerve fibres in epidermis and dermis is four metres per square centimetre.

In the embryo, both the epidermis and the whole nervous system develop from the germ layer known as the ectoderm; their common origin explains the relationship. The position of the nerve endings in layers of the epidermis where vitality is distinctly reduced points to hidden connections which will be considered later.

Sensory perception by the free nerve endings with their organic powers of destruction represents more the death pole in the epidermis. The opposite to this is the metabolism in which pigment-producing cells, or melanocytes, build up pigments in the lowest, more vital zone of the epidermis. These cells have migrated there from the neural crest,

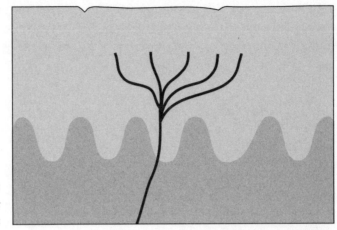

Nerve fibres in the epidermis

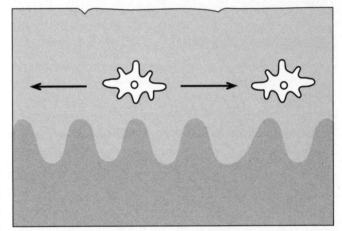

Pigment-producing cells in the epidermis

precursor of the spinal marrow, in the third month of embryonic development. They remain mobile for the whole of a person's life and are constantly on the move among the young horn cells to provide them with the pigment for tanning.

One pigment-producer cell provides for 30 horn cells. The pigment is positioned in the part above their nucleus which is closest to the surface, that is, facing the sun, providing a regular sun screen. The genetic material in the nucleus is thus protected from the UV part of sunlight which could damage it.

In the lower layers of the epidermis are defence cells. Their task is to perceive foreign matter coming in from outside and convey the information to parts of the immune system that are positioned more deeply inside. The organism may then take defensive measures. The distinction between foreign and not foreign thus starts in the epidermis.

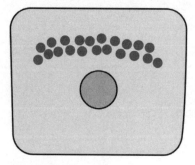

Horn cell with pigment   *Interlinkage of epidermis and dermis*

The dermis or corium

When animal hides are made into leather, the epidermis, hair and all adhering parts of the subcutis are removed, leaving just the dermis. Tanning precipitates the dermal proteins and preserves them. Epidermis and dermis are intensively interlinked, with peglike outgrowths of young horn cells interlinking with convex parts of the dermis. This upper limit to the dermis with its regular wavy lines has a very good blood supply. The convex parts rising from the dermis are called papillae. They contain blood vessels which, coming as arteries from the heart, transport blood to the tip of the papilla; as veins they then take the blood back to the inner body again, towards the heart. The red blood in those vessels shines through the epidermis. The skin is therefore pink where the blood supply is good, and pale when blood withdraws from the periphery to the centre of the organism. The capillary vessels found in one square centimetre of skin have a combined length of about a metre. The capillaries provide all the nutrients and material for the epidermis.

In the papillae and at their lowest boundary, sensory cells serve to perceive various sensory qualities. The structure of these cells, seen not only under a light microscope but in much greater magnification under an electron microscope, is like a bag containing a tall stack of sliced cheese or ham. A tremendous number of fine membranes lie in these

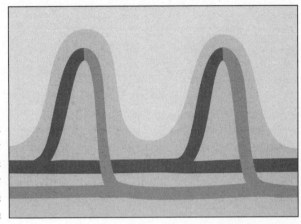

Papillae with capillaries. Left: arterial blood rich in oxygen (dark); right: venous blood low in oxygen

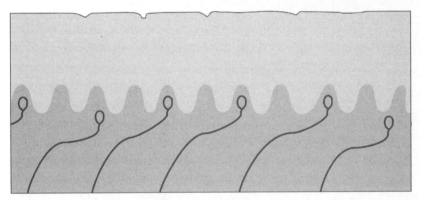

Sensory cells in the upper dermis

cells. Sensory perception is made possible by the stacking of membranes, surfaces and boundaries, which potentiates their effect, as it were.

The dermis is filled from top to bottom with a mesh of fibres of variable elasticity and solidity, and has a mucilaginous (slimy) ground substance which is a solution of proteins, sugars and salts, its composition and reactivity showing much the same uniformity in the organism as a whole as do blood and lymph. Fibres and ground substance provide a framework to hold the various structures in the dermis. The ground substance gives skin its vital fluid tension (turgor), the felted fibres firmness to cope with mechanical stress. The sensory cells are more in the upper zone of the dermis, as stated above; sweat

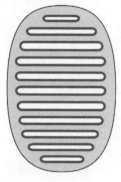

Sensory cells seen under an electron microscope

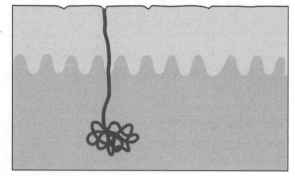

Sweat gland

glands, sebaceous glands and hair follicles lie in the deepest zone, on the border to the subcutis. The production of glandular secretions and of hair is also located down there.

Sweat glands have a sweat-producing lower part, which is a long tube loosely bunched in a ball; the release duct winds its way to the skin surface like a corkscrew. Many different substances are eliminated in the sweat, including salts that make up 0.2–0.3% of sweat. The function of eliminating metabolic products gives sweat glands a certain similarity to the kidneys. Sweat contains all the compounds found in urine, though in low concentration. The cooling effect of sweat evaporating on the skin also regulates body temperature. Nerve impulses govern the secretion of sweat. The distribution of sweat glands varies from area to area. On the back there are 55, on the belly 155, in the palms 375–425, and inside the elbows no less than 751 per square centimetre.

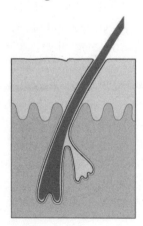

Sebaceous gland

Compared to this, there are only 15 sebaceous glands per square centimetre. Their secretions reach the surface via the hair follicles. Each follicle has its own sebaceous gland. Sebum spreads on the skin surface like oil, sharing the function of protecting the skin with the fat lamellae. The effect of male hormones increases sebum production; this is not only so for men but may also be the case in women if the relative proportions of female to male hormones change. The sebaceous glands relate to the liver, in a way, which also has intensive secretory functions, producing bile. The liver is also the central organ in fat metabolism.

The third kind of glands in the skin are scent glands. Relatively few of them exist, in the underarm areas, around the nipples and in the genital region. The 'scent' is affected by bacterial decomposition of glandular secretions; this is also the case with sweat glands. The well-known body odour often develops when nerves are tense, less so with physical exertion. Today body odour is reduced by showering too often and using synthetic perfumes. The price to be paid for this is quite often dry eczema and allergies.

The ducts coming from all those glands open in our pores. These are visible to the naked eye on the face, but can barely be spotted in other parts of the body. Large pores in the face indicate intense activity of the sebaceous glands which lie closer together in the face and in the hairy scalp. Pores mainly serve to eliminate substances, but the skin can also take up substances through them. Every pore breaks through the barrier of the skin, and substances can enter deeply, going against the flow of secretions. The hairy scalp has particularly many hair follicles, with intake of substances high in that area. This can be utilized, for instance, by applying conditioner to the scalp to nourish the hair.

The realization that the epidermis does not provide a full barrier against substances entering from outside has only come in recent years. Today this openness is utilized by letting medicines enter into the organism via the skin. Examples are hormone patches for post-menopausal women, nicotine patches for giving up smoking, and nitroglycerine patches for people with angina. Recently a gel has come on the market which provides the female body with synthetic hormones.

The possibility of substance being taken in through the skin can also have seriously negative consequences. It has been known to happen when old people applied ointments containing medicinal substances (non-steroidal anti-inflammatory drugs) to painful joints for quite long periods. Long-term use led to serious kidney damage. It must therefore always be remembered that anything applied to the skin can also prove a problem for the organism.

Finally the hair and nails, known as 'skin appendages', are also located in the dermis.

Hair grows from a root supplied with blood and nerves and pushes its way to the surface through the follicle. Under the microscope one can admire the elegant curve in which the hair shaft moves purposefully to the skin surface. The hair on our head grows fastest (0.35 mm/day). The fine body hair grows much more slowly, and the slowest growth is in the eyebrows (0.16 mm/day). A 'good head of hair' immediately shows us that someone is fit and well. We can also see a definite similarity between sprouting hair and the way plants grow. With fingernails and toenails we can say that they also show the fitness and metabolic powers of an organism. Fingernails grow 0.086 mm a day; toenails are definitely slower, with 0.004 mm a day. Hair and nails are another part of the human body that is turning into dead matter, similar to skin scales, though they clearly stay with the body for much longer.

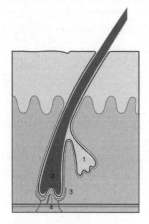

Hair

1 sebaceous gland | 2 hair root | 3 nerves | 4 blood vessels

The subcutis

The inmost layer usually considered to be part of the skin is the subcutis. It is more or less full of fatty tissue, which serves to define the body form. Women have softer, more rounded forms than men. The subcutis also protects bones and internal organs from impact. The fat is really stored heat, and there is some justification in speaking of energy reserves in the fatty tissues of the subcutis.

These reserves are often too large, however, as people tend to overeat today. This excess – it need not always be 10–20 kg, sometimes 3 or 4 kg above a person's normal weight will suffice – provides excessive potential for the generation of heat. Heat roaming through the organism can mean a tendency to develop inflammation, and vital processes may be prevented from taking their normal course in various parts of the body. Both these things can increase the tendency to develop particular skin conditions.

Compared to terrestrial mammals, subcutaneous fatty tissue is well developed in humans. The hippopotamus is an extreme example from the animal world. Well rounded, it nevertheless does not have a layer of fat under the skin, and the flesh in the rest of the body is also low in fat. The creature is thus well adapted to the hot African climate, but it is also tied to it. Human beings are more independent of their environment because they can convert fat into body heat at any time.

Summary: Anatomy of the skin

The skin is seen as having three layers – the epidermis, which produces horn cells, the elastic dermis, which is able to resist mechanical stress, and the subcutis, which stores fat and provides padding and body warmth.

Epidermis and dermis are separated by a basal membrane. The extremely vital epithelial cells which are continually dividing and producing horn cells sit on this. They are provided with the substances they need for survival via the fine capillaries in the upper dermis. Maturing horn cells migrate towards the surface, die off and make up the horny layer. The dead cells are shed from this as skin scales. Horn and fat protect the largely hairless human body skin from outside influences. Urea regulates water metabolism in the horny layer; too little urea causes the skin to dry out. Nerve endings extend as far as the middle of the horny layer, within fractions of millimetres of the skin surface. Pigment-producing cells colour horn cells brown. Defence cells report the presence of foreign invaders.

The interface between epidermis and dermis shows the 'pegs and sockets' of papillae. Sensory cells are concentrated in these, i.e. mainly in the upper layer of the dermis. Sweat glands, sebaceous glands and hair roots, on the other hand, are in the lowest layer, on the boundary to the subcutis. The pores are openings for secretions from sweat, sebaceous and scent glands. Hair and nails, known as skin appendages, are also located in the dermis.

The subcutis consists mostly of fatty tissue and thus serves to shape body form. Fat is stored heat; there is thus some justification in speaking of subcutaneous fat as energy reserves.

The skin and the fourfold human being

This, then, is the anatomy of the skin as seen under the microscope. Much can be learned from it, but it is like a snapshot. When it comes to the sequence of events and to changes in time, it merely depicts a moment.

We see this in a plant. It only reveals its true nature when we have come to know it throughout the year, at the different stages of germination, shooting and sprouting, flowering, fruiting and withering as well as the resting stage in the seed. It is also important to consider the plant's environment, for its form is modified in a damp valley bottom or on light-filled mountain heights. The skin must also be considered in a more comprehensive and dynamic way. Isolated analysis of the organ will not throw any light on the skin's relationship to the organism as a whole.

The question as to powers active in the skin that give rise to its physical condition has not been answered. The skin is not simply a 'sausage skin' (apologies to vegetarians for using this analogy) which covers the body, holding it together. People do ask themselves how soul quality comes to expression in and through the skin, and how human existence in mind and spirit shows itself. In medicine based on natural science it is not possible to answer this question, nor do people want to do so. But these questions are justifiable, as we can certainly see when someone with a severe skin condition comes and asks: Why me? What does this have to do with me? Or questions are asked with regard to healthy skin: Why is my hair fair or dark? Why do I have so many naevi?

To come closer to an answer to these questions we have to look for ideas that do justice to the many different levels of human nature. This will enable us to add to the natural-scientific findings that relate only to the physical aspect. Anthroposophy, established by Rudolf Steiner (1861–1925), proves to be an inexhaustible source of wisdom-filled insight which allows us to solve the problem of the limits set to natural science. Some important ideas in the anthroposophical view of the human being will therefore be given below. Everything said about skin health and diseases in this book is based on these ideas. The author hopes that the book will make it possible for readers to see how modern medicine can be fruitfully broadened by bringing in the holistic anthroposophical approach.

The holistic view of the human being in anthroposophy

For millennia, humanity maintained the link between the higher self and its divine origin. It is only in our present time that the spiritual nature of man has become a question due to a materialistic way of thinking where it is believed that all higher levels of human existence can be shown to arise from material functions. One basic scientific approach based on this view is reductionism where the human being, endowed with mind and spirit, is said to have evolved from a highly developed animal; animals, which have souls, are said to derive from plants with highly complex functions, and living plants from a differentiated physical mechanism. Religion and natural science have thus grown apart from each other in our civilization. And the arts, which really demand insight into the true nature of man, have also lost touch with religion and science. Yet there is a longing felt by every human being to understand his own nature and to know the divine element in the world.

Anthroposophy can meet this basic desire in a way that is right for people of today. It provides insights into inmost human nature and the divine and spiritual nature of the universe. Man and world are shown to have evolved together. From that shared evolution comes the possibility for using substances from the mineral, plant and animal worlds in human medicine, for the processes in human beings and in nature are of the same kind.

The wisdom of all the ancient civilizations may be found in anthroposophy. It has not simply been adopted, however, but newly developed in Rudolf Steiner's spiritual-scientific investigations. Modern people with their natural-scientific education will thus be able to take it in. At the same time it will be possible for people today to go through inner development, develop their powers of insight, and so

17

gain the insights given in anthroposophy for themselves. Anthroposophical inner development leads to powers of soul and organs of perception which will make the spiritual reality that lies beyond sensory perception accessible.

The anthroposophical view of man and world has led to practical initiatives in many spheres of life. Medicine, pharmaceutics, agriculture (biodynamic), education (Waldorf) in kindergartens and schools, curative education, social therapy, fine arts, architecture, speech art, eurythmy, banking and associative forms of economic life have all been given new impulses out of anthroposophy.

The aim of anthroposophical medicine is not only to provide comprehensive treatment for the sick, with consultation, medicaments, external applications, art and eurythmy therapies. It is also to enable patients to take their situation in hand themselves. Deeper understanding of health, sickness and healing enables them to take the initiative and consciously work towards their own health. The holistic approach to medicine broadened through anthroposophy can thus encourage personal responsibility.

Tension exists between the analytical (considering the parts) process, where one goes into detail, and the synthesizing (bringing things together) approach, where the living organism is seen as a whole. Thinking of how to overcome this, the German writer Goethe wrote:

To delight in the whole,
look for that whole in even the smallest part.

Below, we will follow this principle in answering the question: How can we see the whole human being reflected in the skin? How does the human being show himself at all the different levels of his existence in the skin?

All things that take material form also have their spiritual and soul aspect. And all things that occur in spirit and soul also have their external, material aspect. Rudolf Steiner

The physical body truly is merely a gesture which points to the true human being. Rudolf Steiner

The level of mind and spirit—the I

Let us begin with the highest level of human existence, which is in the spirit. It provides the opportunity for every human being on earth to be a unique individual (indivisible). Existence in the spirit makes it possible to have one's own, wholly individual biography.

It is existence in the spirit which makes human beings human, and awareness into self-awareness. We call this spiritual principle which each has for his own the self or 'I'. What enables the I to live in the body? The warmth that is present throughout the body. We may speak of a 'warmth organism' which generates its own heat, with differentiated regions of warmth and areas where temperatures are lower. The movement of the blood gives the warmth organism the power to move within itself, for instance to keep hands and feet warm on a cold winter's day. We are thus able to say that the human I lives in the warmth of the blood and can see this particularly well when someone 'warms to a thought'. Enthusiasm for an idea brings him alive, the skin grows pink and he warms up from top to toe.

In the skin we thus find the spiritual aspect in the blood. A fright or fear of something makes us go pale; the I withdraws before the world together with the blood. It is different with the blush of embarrassment. Confronted with something we have said or done, we may feel that our inner nature has been laid bare, and the I wants to hide behind the blood. The human I thus has a powerful influence on the blood, and the best way of telling how some news affects a person is to observe the way the colour changes in the face. We generally tend to do this, though in a wholly unconscious way.

The anatomical site for this I-activity in the skin is that of the capillaries in the papillae of the upper dermis.

The effect of the I on the finest blood vessels in the skin is thus immediately apparent to others. It is different with another important site of I-activity which lies hidden deep down in the subcutaneous fatty tissue of the subcutis. Fat serves the I in that it is able to generate heat. With the aid of its fats, the organism is a self-contained heat system independent of the environment. This gives human beings the freedom to live in different climates.

Ultimately the whole skin with all its layers is formed out by the human I so that the body may be an instrument for the I. 'In human

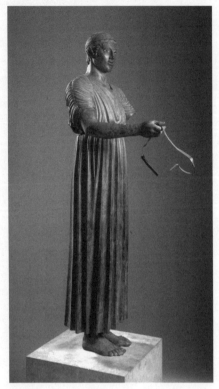

The Charioteer at Delphi

beings, it is above all the organs that lie in the periphery of the body which are penetrated and configured by the I' (Rudolf Steiner). This is also why we identify so strongly with our skin. It is important to us, and even a minor change in it makes us ask for medical advice from a skin specialist. The genius of language lets the skin stand for the whole human being. 'Getting away with a whole skin' means that the whole person gets out of the situation unharmed. The skin represents all four levels of human existence and also the conditions under which we live on earth, having been born into them thanks to destiny.

The level of the soul

Human beings live with their I embedded in the soul level of existence. They have soul in common with the animal world. Both humans and animals are ensouled. Animals live in their reflexes and species-specific behaviour patterns. The I living in the human soul makes it possible to kindle the light of thought, to know good from evil in a life of free thought.

Looking for the physical location where the psyche is most active, we come to the nerves. The nervous system makes the human organism come awake and gives conscious awareness of the body. The sense organs, which arise from the nerves, perceive the world around us, above all the light and the environment given lustre by the light. The light-filled airy atmosphere gives the most life to the soul, for we take in light through the gateways of the senses and air into the organism through the lungs.

In the skin, nerves supply mainly the epidermis and upper dermis, allowing us to react quickly or more slowly. You may be said to have a thick or a thin skin. Nerves can be over-tense, react too soon or for too long; the skin may have too much conscious awareness, be too awake, as in the case of pruritus (itching). We get 'goose pimples' when we hear something unpleasant. A muscle in the upper dermis which serves to make hair come upright is stimulated by the nerve and contracts; the epidermis close to the hair then rises in a small cone.

Animal skin can also reflect emotions. If a dog or cat gets frightened, for example, the hair along the spine stands upright like a brush. An animal cannot grow pale or blush, however, and even if it could this would not be visible through the hair or fur. Animals can also be warm-blooded, but they lack the connection between I and blood system

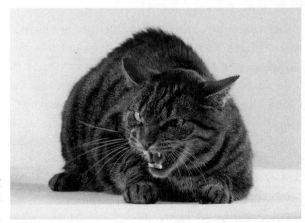

Hair growing along the spine comes upright like a brush

21

which is characteristic of humans. The distinct relationship between human beings and higher vertebrates indicates that thanks to a common evolution, animals are orientated towards man.

The level of life

The level of vitality, of vital processes, which we share with the plant world, may also be found in the skin. In the human organism, vital energies are most actively involved in anabolism (constructive metabolism). The best example of this is the liver with its immense metabolism and powers of regeneration. 'Liver' and 'live' are clearly related, with the liver the absolute site of life.

In the skin, vital processes are concentrated in the production of glandular secretions and in hair and nail growth. Continuous cell division in the lowest layer of the epidermis also shows that there is vitality there, but this is balanced out by the early death process of horn cells. Cell regeneration has to be active in this area so that the epidermis, our boundary with the outside world, will survive under all conditions in life. It must not happen, for instance, that a long period of hard work in the garden completely wears away the epidermis on the palms. On the other hand, regeneration, skin vitality, also must not go beyond certain limits; the human skin must not have so much life and powers of growth that we develop a shell like that of a tortoise or a pelt like that of a bear. Here the powers of the I intervene, limiting and regulating skin vitality so that it does not go beyond the human level.

The vital production of glandular secretions is followed by a second step, which is secretion and elimination through the pores in the skin surface. Once again the human psyche comes into play. Sweat and sebaceous (or oil) glands are supplied with nerves. Certain emotions cause increased glandular secretion. When we are tense before an examination, for example, we tend to sweat more in the palms and under our arms. Smokers quite often produce more sebum, for nicotine creates a situation in the organism where smokers may feel a degree of euphoria. Such feelings go hand in hand with increased sebum production, and it is not uncommon for smokers to have shiny faces.

The physical level

We find the purely physical level of human existence in the stream of nutrients, in the transport of substances from one site to another to maintain the form of the physical body. This physical level exists also in the skin. The stream of matter comes to the skin from inside, moving to the outside, passing centrifugally through all skin layers and organs.

This produces the physical skin with its tissues and cells. It is composed to suit the human individual who lives in it. This means that the human I is active even at the physical level of existence, configuring the skin down to the smallest detail. There must not be any skin process where the I does not take a hand. A brief example is this. In the epidermis, isolated pigment-producing cells appear among the mass of horn cells in the lowest layer, and isolated defence cells occur in the layer above. Both cell types are evenly distributed in the epidermis. In the third month of embryonic development, the pigment cells migrate from the neural tube, the precursor of the bone marrow, to the epidermis, and their path from the back to the front in the dermis is a long one. The defence cells move centrifugally from the precursor of the bone marrow to the epidermis via the blood from the fifth month onwards. The directions taken by pigment cells and defence cells do thus cross. And the functions of the two cell types also cross. Pigment cells are nerve cells by origin. They function as unicellular glands, however, and are full of pigment-producing metabolic processes. The defence cells originate in the blood and develop sensory functions in the skin, for they can identify foreign matter. One cell thus moves from nervous system to metabolism, the other from the blood, instrument for metabolism, to a sensory function which relates to the nervous system.

Sublime wisdom coming from the human I lies in these subtle physical processes. With the threefold crossover which I have described, the skin as the largest sense organ subconsciously bears the signature of something which we must today, in our culture, develop as an ability by consciously working on our own powers of sensory perception. The dogma of modern science is that we must refrain from making our own judgement when obtaining research data. An important example of this is the double-blind trial method in demonstrating medicinal actions. Neither physician nor patient knows if the actual medicine or a placebo is being given or taken. In exactly the opposite way, a scientist who has trained his sensory perceptions and gained new skills will be able to perceive the wisdom that lies behind a natural process. He uses his will to transform his powers of perception so that the divine wisdom reveals itself as he observes the world around him. In the words of Rudolf Steiner this means that 'human will' and 'world thoughts' meet. Self awareness arises at the point where they meet and the eye is opened for the spirit which lies behind all outward existence. 'We need an inner attitude where we are truly, at any moment of our waking life, aware of the principles which our higher senses show us to be at work in our immediate surroundings' (Rudolf Steiner). The above-mentioned threefold crossover is like a faculty that lies dormant in us and must be taken up with some energy.

Summary: The skin and the fourfold human being

The organization of the human being thus creates its own outer limits in the skin at all four levels of essential human nature — the spiritual through the blood system, soul quality through the nervous system, life in the development of glands, hair and nails, and at the physical and material level with the transport of matter which comes to a halt in the skin. This is the deeper reason for the complicated anatomy of the skin, an organ which reflects the many-layered nature of the human being. We may compare it to a complex natural textile where sheep's wool, silk, cotton and linen are interwoven. But it is the spirit in the human being, the I, which guides the process, creating a reflection of itself at the levels of soul, life and physical existence.

This can be shown in tabular form as follows.

Level of existence	Element	Organ in the skin	Skin layer
spirit (I)	warmth	blood	upper dermis
soul	light, air	nerve	epidermis, upper dermis
life	fluid	gland	lower dermis
physical	solid matter	all-present	whole skin

The skin and the threefold human being

The four levels of human existence can also be seen as pairs of opposites, with spirit and soul serving conscious life in the waking soul, and the living physical body providing the material basis for this. Spirit and soul come to expression in the physical body, revealing themselves with the aid of it.

At this point we may ask how spirit and soul work together with the living body. This is the key question in psychosomatic medicine, concerning the interaction between psyche and soma (body). The idea of the threefold organism proves extraordinarily helpful in finding an answer. Rudolf Steiner introduced this as part of his anthroposophical anthropology in 1917, having sought it for 30 years following his schooldays. The idea is described below and related to the skin.

The neurosensory system

The nervous system and sense organs are a functional whole which is located mainly in the region of the human head. This is where the most important sense organs are, above all eye and ear, sense of balance, taste and smell. The largest sense organ in anatomical terms is the skin, however, with its sense of touch and the ability to perceive temperature differences, pain and pressure.

The neurosensory system serves the waking, conscious life of the soul. Different sensory qualities bring the outside world into the human organism. Anything perceived is taken in and digested in thought. Thinking at soul level is organically bound to nerve functions.

Activity in the neurosensory system is always connected with destructive processes. An example is the breakdown of visual purple in the retina of the eye under the influence of light. The visual purple is a pigment in the sensory cells of the eye; perception only becomes possible when it breaks down. The sensory cells are not themselves able to synthesize new visual purple; this needs the blood's powers of providing nourishment.

Nerve function is cooling. It is not for nothing that we speak of the 'cool head' needed in difficult situations. In a 'cool type', sensory perception and rapid reaction function well, a characteristic of modern people in the western world, who live so much in their nerves and senses that they tend to be one-sided.

Essentially, all activity in nerves and senses depends on an outwardly resting state. The head must be in calm balance so that we may 'keep our heads'. When someone is in a rage, a tremendous urge to move has overpowered the calm region of the human being's nerves and senses. Concussion caused by a blow to the head, for instance, also upsets the resting state of the brain so much that the individual loses consciousness for a moment. He will then no longer remember what happened immediately before the blow was struck, which is one sign on which the diagnosis of concussion is based.

At the organic level, powers to give form and differentiate are connected with nerve function. If we look at the human form it is immediately obvious that in the upper pole, in the face, form is so marked that it makes us unique individuals. It would not be so easy to identify someone by their belly or behind, where rounded forms show less differentiation.

Much of the skin thus serves the neurosensory system. Nerves and sensory cells in the epidermis and upper dermis take conscious awareness to the body's boundaries, make the skin be awake and so the organism as a whole open to sensory perception of the environment. The destructive processes and differentiation connected with nerve function at the organic level can be seen in the death of horn cells in the epidermis and their biochemical differentiation as horn substance and fat lamellae mature, for the close proximity between free nerve endings and horn cells suggests that it is the nervous system with its particular laws which is responsible for what happens to the horn cells.

Metabolism and limbs

The polar opposite of the neurosensory system is the metabolic system, which is mainly located in the abdomen. In the limbs, the internal mobility of metabolism comes together with external mobility. In health, all metabolic activity is unconscious, that is, in a sleep state. It needs a pathological disorder such as gastric (stomach) pains to wake an organ up and come to conscious awareness. In that case, powers of soul no longer 'breathe' in the organ concerned, and intestinal move-

26

ment may slow down, for instance. Those powers then connect too strongly with the living physical body and spasmodic pain develops.

Organically, the main activity of metabolism is to build up substance and serve regeneration. The blood takes this activity to all areas of the body. We can see that the human being of nerves and the human being of metabolism interpenetrate; it would be wrong and utterly schematic to think of one being located wholly in the upper and the other wholly in the lower body. The blood takes not only constructive powers through the organism but also heat. Good food warms, and so does physical labour. With the latter, and the flowing of the juices and a metabolism of constant mixing, merging and interacting, we have movement as the opposite to the calm in the human being of nerves. Where a nervous impulse creates form and differentiated configuration, metabolism fills these with substance.

In the skin, metabolic activity is most intensive and varied in the lower dermis where glandular secretions, hair and nails are produced. The skin contains about 300,000 sebaceous glands which together release 2 or 3 g of sebum per day; 2 million sweat glands produce $\frac{1}{2}$ litre of sweat a day without the individual being aware of sweating. Major physical effort and a warm environment can increase the volume to as much as 10 litres a day. The hair on the head grows 1 mm in three days, and a fingernail 1 mm in 12 days on average. These are some of the measurable effects which metabolism has in the skin, showing the skin to be not only a sense organ but also a site for metabolism.

Another site for metabolism in the skin is the fat tissue in the subcutis. We can best see what happens there if we compare subcutis and epidermis, as follows.

With numerous round fat cells showing monotony of form in the subcutis, the epidermis is distinctly stratified, its horn cells hexagonal. The subcutis is relatively thick — millimetres to centimetres — whereas the epidermis is extremely thin at 75 micrometres to a maximum of half a millimetre. It looks as if a powerful form principle has flattened it out, rather like a flake of gold used for gilding. Ongoing metabolism is dominant in the subcutis. Fat newly taken up by the intestines is channelled towards the fat cell via the blood and deposited there. Fat stored in fat tissue is mobilized and made available to the internal organs as needed. Fat thus serves metabolism. The substances in the epidermis, on the other hand, serve mainly to build up horny substance in the horn cells and fat lamellae between the cells. These substances are kept in place, maintaining the epidermis's barrier function, for a short period before leaving the skin as scales, 'fodder' for dust mites. This comparison between subcutis and epidermis shows how closely the fat tissue in the subcutis is connected with metabolism in the human organism as a whole.

We use our limbs to implement our plans. Thought is followed by will impulse and then action. This means that the part of our inner life by which we connect with the world is very much bound up with metabolism and limbs. In anthroposophical anthropology the soul level is thus considered to relate to the body in a differentiated way. Nerves and senses are merely the place where thinking evolves. Activity arising from the will, on the other hand, has its sphere of action in metabolism and limbs.

In modern psychology, it is too often thought that the seat of the soul is in the head, the brain, only. This wrong idea has found general acceptance as may be seen from the way in which people tend to point a finger at the forehead when someone whose soul quality they don't understand has annoyed them. This would be more meaningful if the thinking had been faulty. In everyday life the opposite is often the case, however, when someone (or oneself) has no proper control over his will impulses. This is always the case when we 'burst a blood vessel'. Anger causes the blood to rise mightily from the lower human being with our will; blood flow to the neck and head increases, filling the vessels to near bursting point. We should really point to people's bellies rather than point a finger at our forehead.

The polarity between neurosensory system on the one hand and metabolism and limbs on the other may be summed up as follows.

Neurosensory system	Metabolism and limbs
waking state, day	sleep, night
nerve	blood
destruction	synthesis
coolness	warmth
at rest	in motion
form	matter
thinking	acting out of the will

In the neurosensory system, the human mind and spirit (the I) and the soul live in loose connection with the living physical basis. The energies released in destructive processes are transformed and taken to the soul level where they serve our thinking. We tend to say that one thought grows from another, having the image of a plant in mind, because we have a feeling for the connection between vital energies and powers of thought. Sensory perception and the digestion of our perceptions as well as the forming of ideas and memory functions are activities in the soul based on the neurosensory system.

In metabolism and limbs, on the other hand, spirit and soul have entered deeply into the physical. The human I fully configures the metabolic organs from within, and the whole locomotor system is also created down to the smallest detail out of the I's powers. Guided by the spiritual level of their existence, human beings build a body for themselves — starting from embryonic development — that is the instrument for bringing individual impulses that are utterly their own to bear in shaping their biography. In the early years of life these developmental processes still extend to the neurosensory system, which is why we cannot remember those years, for instance. In the microcosm of our internal organs, matter we have taken in is subject to impulses given by the I and broken down completely in the digestive processes of the intestines. It is then made into the body's own substance by being given life in the liver and soul under the influence of the kidney, and is filled with spirit and made truly human thanks to the activity of the heart.

If we had to live solely in the polarity of neurosensory system on the one hand and metabolism and limbs on the other, we would either consume ourselves in nervous, excessive wakefulness or drown in the dim unconscious state of metabolism. A third element is needed for the human organization, to balance out extremes and create harmony between nerve and blood. This has been given to us in rhythm.

The rhythmical system

Life can only unfold in the to and fro between sleep and waking, work and periods of relaxation, sensory perception and reflection, inhalation and exhalation, diastole (relaxation of the heart) and systole (contraction of the heart). The rhythmical system provides the mediating middle between the upper and lower systems.

The rhythmical system has its main location in the chest region of the human form, where heart and lung have their seat. Breath and pulse go through the whole human being, however. Sensory perception is possible only in the alternation between taking things in whilst wide awake and working them through inwardly in our thinking.

This also casts some light on the way the skin breathes. Being a sense organ, the skin alternates between being open, ready to receive, and being closed up, insensitive. The breathing of the skin, as it is commonly called, does not compare with the breathing of the lungs. The skin only takes in 1.9% of the oxygen and gives off 2.7% of the carbon dioxide converted in the organism as a whole. The 'breathing of the skin' refers more to giving off sweat which evaporates on the skin surface and the reception of sensory stimuli. For both it is best to wear airy clothing made from natural materials.

Feeling is the element in the life of the soul that corresponds to the to and fro between nerve and blood, between thinking and acting out of the will. We warm to a thought in our feelings and are then able to use the will to bring it to realization. Our feeling thus mediates between thinking and doing, which makes this sphere a special field of activity for the human I. We sometimes say something is 'close to my heart'. The central organ of the rhythmical system is seen as the place where we cherish things that are particularly dear or important to us. And things we 'take to heart' are given very special consideration. We 'take heart' when we show courage. But when the heart 'goes down to one's boots' the head produces possible objections and we cannot bring the will and our desire for action to bear. The phrase 'with all one's heart and soul' occurs repeatedly in the Bible. The genius of language shows that higher powers can arise in the middle human being from a Christian spirit and give us strength and courage for everyday life and work.

In the skin, the rhythmical system is most concentrated in the upper dermis. Blood rhythmically flows to and from the fine capillaries. We have already referred to the rhythm of sensory perception in the skin and above all in the sensory cells in the upper dermis. The free nerve endings serving the sense of touch in the epidermis are more uninterrupted in their function. This is also why we can wake someone up during the night by touching them.

We have thus found threefold human nature in soul, function and anatomy to exist also in the skin. There is a region in the skin which is rather like the head. Its opposite is a layer where metabolism predominates. Between them lies a zone which is specifically connected with the rhythmical system. With all three systems thus represented, we may call the skin a universal organ. All spheres of the organism are reflected in the skin, and this means that the skin is also connected with the different regions of the body and interactions take place in all areas.

With the skin as threefold as the whole organism, health and disease in the skin must be connected with a particular personality type. Skin diseases where function tends to be one-sided are described in the next chapter. Considering the connections between body and soul it is possible to add particular personality traits to many of the descriptions of particular skin conditions, where thinking, feeling and acting out of the will act together in a way typical of the given condition. One can actually say that when knowledge of the skin has been broadened in this way it is possible to gain self-knowledge by observing specific inherited, constitutional skin characteristics.

Summary: The skin and the threefold human being

The idea of the threefold nature of the human organism casts light on the interaction between soul and body. Soul life can be considered in a differentiated way in relation to the three regions of the body. Thinking

System	main anatomical site	inner activity	site in the skin
Neurosensory system	head – above	thinking	epidermis
Rhythmical system	chest – middle	feeling	upper dermis
Metabolism and limbs	abdomen – below	doing	lower dermis, subcutis

is made possible because we have nerves and senses, feeling because of our rhythmical middle, and the will to act through metabolism and limbs.

This may be shown in tabular form (see previous page).

The skin in the field of tension between matter and form

Having considered the activities of fourfold human nature and the concept of the threefold human organism with reference to the skin, we will now try a third way of doing justice to the different aspects of the skin in all its complex structure.

Differences and effects of the powers of matter and of form

The creation and maintenance of an organ with its internal structure and outer form can be compared to the work of a sculptor. The relative proportions of water and fine-grained solid matter give his material, perhaps a lump of clay, a certain weight, a degree of softness and plasticity. This clay is one component in the evolving work of art. It lies on the bench, heavy, shapeless and occupying space. The artist's powers of imagination have put a particular form before his inner eye. The hand, especially the fingertips, give the clay that form; this is the second component.

The sculpture arises as the artist applies powers of form under the guidance of his inner image. These powers act towards a central point from the periphery. The space-occupying power of the material opposes them; its direction of action is from centre to periphery. The sensitive interaction between powers of matter and of form — and the artist must take them into account — is easily disrupted. He may be upset, suffer from lack of

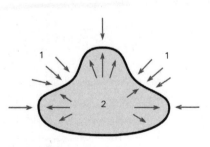

Power of form (1) and matter (2)

32

sleep or have had a drop to drink — any of this may make the artistic process impossible. The sculpture is then deformed. Disruption may of course also come from the material; the clay may be too wet, for example, and collapse upon itself.

The situation is very similar with the powers active in the organs of the human body. The skin, too, is under the influence of powers of matter and form. The substances that make up the skin and regenerate its structures come from the blood, which moves from centre to periphery. We may speak of a living centrifugal stream of matter coming to the skin with the blood, going beyond its boundaries in form of glandular secretions, hair and nails as well as dandruff and skin flakes. Part of the stream is taken in another direction, however, and goes back to the centre, to the heart. The reversal of flow comes in the capillaries of the papillae; the tip of every papilla presents the image of the curve which is followed by the stream of matter in changing direction.

It is interesting to learn from the anthroposophical study of man that a change in the direction in which streams of matter flow is connected with coming to conscious awareness. Two examples: Walking in the dark, we bump into a hard object. The part of the body with which we do so, its movement stopped by the object, feels pain. The degree of conscious awareness has increased abruptly in this part. Taking a shower that ends with alternating hot and cold has a similar effect, though this is felt to be pleasant. Blood flow increases in the skin and therefore also the reversal of flow in the capillaries. This makes us feel really good in our bodies.

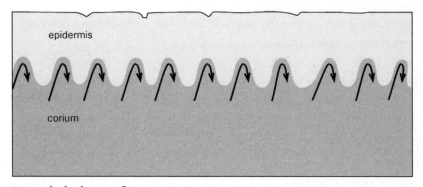

Reversal of substance flow

The powers of matter are opposed by powers of form which set boundaries and configure forms. The skin is certainly not just an outer covering, as is evident from the fact that in embryonic development the impulse to develop an arm or a leg comes from the skin. A fold develops, a bud, with internal differentiation of tissues following. The powers of form are most active in the epidermis. We have seen that the epidermis is in the widest sense responsible for creating barriers against foreign matter. It also develops form-giving activity in the depths of the dermis. Sebaceous and sweat glands, hair follicle and nail-generating organ are really created by the epidermis going deep down into the dermis to develop the organs it needs for glandular functions and the growth of hair and nails. These are then taken hold of by the constructive powers of metabolism so that secretions and skin appendages may be synthesized. Form and matter thus work together.

If we consider the epidermis on its own with reference to the activities of the two powers, we find that the above-mentioned polarity exists here as well. In the lowest layer, cell bodies are round, filled with fluid, thus showing vitality and plasticity. They are also capable of division. In the superficial horny layer, on the other hand, cells are flat, like roof tiles, dry, often bizarre shapes, and dead. In the lower layer of the epidermis living powers of matter are dominant, in the upper layer powers of form that kill off life.

Powers of matter come to the fore in the places where the body surface turns inward and then changes to a moist mucosa (mucous membrane). They are particularly active in the intestinal mucosa, causing new cells to develop all the time, as old ones are shed, so that stools consist to a large part of dead cells. This, and the mucosa's marked ability to produce secretions from its glands, sometimes in large quantities, shows that there is a tendency to dissolve. The upper layers of the epidermis on the other hand show hardening processes. Working with gardening tools, for instance, produces calluses in the areas of the palm where mechanical stress is greatest; solid, hard areas where the skin has thickened. Hair and nails also show that tendency to harden, a sign that powers of form are particularly active.

Transition from the phenomena described for the healthy epidermis to symptoms of skin disease is gradual. Pathological tendencies arise from activities of opposing powers which in themselves are healthy. If powers of hardening go beyond a certain limit, pathological cornification and sclerosis develop. If the powers that soften tissue and cause cell growth take the upper hand, the skin will tend to get inflamed.

Where do those powers of form come from? One thing we can see directly is that sunlight has powerful form-giving effects on skin that has been exposed to it for a whole life. It is mainly the ultraviolet part of sunlight which thins the connective tissue in the dermis and so makes the skin flaccid and wrinkled. Country people and seafarers have such suntanned skin full of wrinkles. Fair-skinned, blue-eyed people may certainly expect to have many wrinkles in old age if they expose themselves a lot to the sun. The skin has another protective mechanism as well as tanning. This is the development of hyperkeratosis (excessive horny growth) caused by light, where the thickness of the callus increases after a few days of exposure to the sun in order to keep out light. This is a constructive activity on the part of the epidermis, but it is triggered by the sun's powers to impose form and to harden. This is an example of form-giving powers from our human environment directly affecting the skin.

A more deep-reaching effect of sunlight is due to vitamin D. This regulates calcium metabolism and calcium deposits in bone, giving it form and stability. Sunlight is needed to differentiate fully functional vitamin D out from a precursor which is a metabolic product in the skin. This can then take the form-giving, stabilizing power of sunlight to the bones in the human body.

When organs develop, the organism's own generative powers are, of course, much more important than outside influences. They are mediated by the nervous system. We have seen that free nerve endings cause horn cells to die off and mature fully. The barrier function, that is, forming a boundary, also depends on regular maturation. Excessive nerve impulses cause excessive form in the skin, weak nerve impulses too much metabolism and a tendency for the skin to get inflamed.

Finally let us consider differences in the skin and in form for people at different ages. In older adults, powers of form have drawn lines in the face based on individual facial expression. The element of spirit and soul has been working on the living body and this has produced a unique face, posture and also gait. With alcoholics, for instance, it is difficult for the spirit and soul to be active, and the subtle, individual nature of facial forms is lost. We can see a wrinkled face as something positive, for it bears the marks of what the individual has thought, felt, gone through and also intended in life. Looking at wrinkles from this point of view, we won't think of using wrinkle-removing creams or getting a face lift. The opposite to this is the skin of an infant. It is smooth, soft, pink, firmly rounded and elastic. Neither sunlight nor individual inner life have left a mark so far.

Summary: The skin in the field of tension between matter and form

Matter and form act in opposition to one another. The flow of matter goes from inside to outside. In the capillaries of the papillae it turns around and flows back to the centre, to the heart. Sunlight provides powers of form from outside. Their more deep-reaching action via vitamin D production supports bone development. The inner powers of form arise from the nervous system.

In the epidermis, the actions of matter and form are evident in the opposition between vitality in the lower zone and death processes, with horn and skin flakes being produced, in the upper zone.

The polarity of matter and form may be summed up as follows.

Powers of matter	Powers of form
lower epidermis	upper epidermis
glands, mucous membrane	calluses, hair, nails
dissolution	hardening
inflammation	sclerosis

Acids protecting the skin

The dead horn cells on the skin surface are wetted with sebum and sweat. Sweat is slightly acid, and sebum contains many fatty acids. In the human organism, acid fluids bear the signature of the neuro-sensory system, basic fluids that of metabolism. This also applies to the skin surface, which is moist with sweat and sebum.

It is currently assumed that the acid on the skin surface is protection against germs. Countless germs live on healthy skin, for a place where living matter from the human organism is about to change into dead matter provides a good nutrient base for them (8 million micro-organisms per square centimetre of skin). The spectrum of germs is comparable in size to that of intestinal microorganisms. The kind and number of individual elements of this skin flora must, however, be within certain limits if it is to keep the skin healthy, working together with the acid sweat and sebum. Washing too frequently with soap or synthetic detergents will destroy the acid protection and healthy microorganisms. The horny layer swells and those detergents may draw fat from even deeper layers, which gives them an even greater drying effect than soaps.

Why are humans naked?

One of the most noticeable characteristics of human skin is its unprotectedness, its nakedness. Human beings do not have fur or feathers, horny plates, spines, quills, horns, manes or a tuft of hair on a tail. Animals have specific skin appendages that enable them to cope with a particular climate, and humans do not have these.

This means, however, that the powers which in animals are needed to make hair and feathers grow become freely available in human beings and can be transformed into powers of thought. Fur, feathers and all other horny skin appendages in the animal world arise from the epidermis, as we have seen. The epidermis is the main site for neurosensory activity, and so it is not difficult to see the connection. In earlier times, feathers were still cut to size and dipped into ink for writing, letting one's thoughts flow into the feather – an expressive image for the connection between thought and feather.

The feathers worn for adornment by North American Indians are of great anthropological interest. The myths of the Indians reflected a most ancient, highly evolved wisdom. Nineteenth-century photographs often show faces revealing great inner maturity. Decorative eagles' feathers, the longest worn in the head region, reflect this. The head-dresses would often extend down as far as the lower leg on both sides, with feathers getting smaller and smaller lower down. This gives us a magnificent image for powers of growth and development that have come free in the human head region so that they can take in wisdom through thought activity. The fact that the feathers get smaller lower down indicates that the powers of growth and development are tied up in the organs in this region of metabolic activity and unconscious will.

Human nakedness has other aspects as well. We have seen how the blood, in which the I lives, and which goes as far as the capillaries in the upper dermis, is visible through the epidermis. This makes it possible to see what is going on in someone. It is only possible where the skin is not covered by hair or pigmented. The blood shining through creates a quite specific colour which is characteristic of human skin. Peach blossom comes closest to it. This colour tone presents a living image of the human I in unpigmented areas. The spirit creates it in the blood's fullness of life. In German this flesh tone is called 'incarnation colour', for the background to it is the human spirit and soul incarnating in the flesh. It tells us something of the individual's inmost nature.

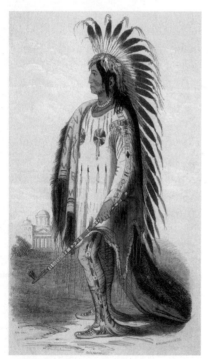

North American Indian wearing feathered headdress of body length, from Catlin, G. Die Indianer Nordamerikas, *Leipzig 1851*

The nakedness of human skin makes it impossible for the organism to create a warm inner space for itself with a hairy pelt or plumage. To make up for this, blood supply to the skin is highly variable, with the skin also able to vary the amount of heat given off via the skin. We have already spoken of the well-developed fatty tissues in the human subcutis. These two factors give the human temperature organization a great degree of freedom and independence. The body is able to maintain its own internal temperature within the skin at a wide range of environmental temperatures. This is interesting if we consider that the human I lives in warmth and communicates with other levels of existence by changing the temperature level. Having his own I, man, the crown of creation, clearly needs to have a much more differentiated way of dealing with temperatures than animals do.

A naked human skin needs to be clothed, and we also need shelter. This calls civilizing powers to life. We may choose different natural materials, dye them, sew different styles, or process them by specific methods to develop different fabrics. This enables human beings to express their individual nature. A free space is given where each can bring in his individual style.

The individual expression shown in the open, non-hairy face thus continues on in our individual choice of clothing. Special garments may be worn on special occasions. In the past, people at a particular level of spiritual development – initiates and priests – wore garments that revealed the special relationship between their existence in spirit and soul on the one hand and in the body on the other. The North American Indian headdress is a simple example of this.

Architecture, which provides us with the necessary shelter, also offers many opportunities to bring spirit and soul into play in shaping our building materials.

Summary: Why are humans naked?

Apart from its protective acids, human skin does not have the additional protection of fur or feather – a challenge to human beings to be free in creating the protection they need through clothing and shelter. Having no need for protective organic appendages, human beings have the powers animals need for these available for their spiritual and mental faculties.

We need to observe
the spiritual in the physical;
this alone will make us understand
the nature of illness.

Rudolf Steiner

SKIN DISEASES

The brief indications given below as to how the causes of skin conditions may lie in metabolism, the psyche or an inherited constitution may help readers to see how complicated and difficult it is for the physician to find the causes in a particular case. This book clearly cannot take the place of a skin specialist. It needs extensive dermatological and general medical training and considerable medical experience to treat skin conditions in anthroposophical medicine.

It is a great help to the physician if patients meet his efforts with some degree of understanding, with an insight into the general situation that is based on sound common sense. This book is intended to create and enhance such insight and understanding.

Causes of skin conditions

A skin condition, be it short-term or long-lasting, perhaps even lifelong, may have all kinds of different causes. There may be a weakness in metabolism, with the liver, kidneys, pancreas or intestine being perfectly healthy but sluggish in the way they function.

A simple comparison will show this. Lazy people may generally be in good organic health, they simply don't do much work. In the same way the liver may be perfectly healthy, with no increase in the level of liver enzymes released into the blood when liver cells break down due to damage done to the organ. In spite of this the liver may have a functional disorder; it is not doing what it should be doing, at least not properly, which means that the skin or other organs have to do these things for it.

The skin, as has been shown, is the universal organ which will then have to deal with disorders of this kind. It has to do work for which it is not designed, and this produces the symptoms of skin disease.

On the other hand, the causes of skin problems may also lie in the psyche. Stress at work when physical defences are low, in winter, for instance, may encourage the development of a skin disorder. Or a sudden event may have come as a shock, and this changes the balance between destructive and constructive metabolism in the skin in the direction of the skin breaking down. Not knowing ourselves and our limits properly may make us do the wrong thing or ask too much of ourselves in social life over and over again. This means stress for mind and nerves, which in turn makes the skin susceptible to certain diseases.

An inherited constitution will often aggravate both the causes that lie in the metabolic sphere and those due to being unable to cope with everyday life. That constitution has been chosen. Prior to conception, the incarnating human being chooses parents with the genetic make-up required for the new life on earth.

One should not imagine this choice to be like going to a store and choosing a suit or a dress. It arises from the wise workings of destiny, a wisdom that will only rarely emerge from the dark depths of the soul in everyday life. At birth, the individual is placed in specific conditions for life. The nature of the physical body is something which is given, and so is a particular kind of skin. The colours of our skin, eyes and hair are fixed for life, and cannot be changed, as is whether our skin is dry or oily. We are also born thin-skinned and sensitive, or thick-skinned, and this is an example of how we also speak of our mental make-up as 'skin'.

Skin disease and yeasts in the intestine

Skin conditions frequently go hand in hand with digestive problems, a good example of interaction between the inner and outer parts of the organism.

With many patients, a skin specialist will also pay special attention to the condition of the intestines and their digestive functions. (In the section on neurodermatitis, a description is given of the connection between this condition and a weak digestion.) People with the four most common skin conditions

- neurodermatitis
- psoriasis
- seborrhoeic dermatitis and
- nettle rash (urticaria)

more often than not have dense yeast populations in the intestine.

How does this happen? What is the connection between two organ systems which are as far apart as intestine and skin?

What those four skin conditions have in common is that an inflammatory process in the organism's periphery is tying up energies. Those energies are then lacking in the inner organism, for instance in the digestion. The result is that the process of breaking down foods is weak. It is, however, essential for foods to be broken down completely so that they may be used to create the body's own substance. Before the body can make something which is foreign its own, all foreign quality must be stripped away. If this is not properly done, the material is still partly foreign and creates the soil in which microorganisms can grow in the intestinal tract. These will flourish at a density that is not right for the human intestine. They are primarily yeasts, especially those of the Candida family.

The gastrointestinal tract is an eco-system where the human being lives together with vast numbers of different microorganisms. Being the host, he provides the soil in which the bacteria live in countless abundance, benefiting the human being in turn. They break down food substances for which the human being has no use, and give off substances into the intestine which serve the human metabolism.

Human infants and young children have to come to terms with this intestinal flora in a process that is most important for developing the immune system. The defence system acts like a gardener in the intestine who makes careful distinction between vegetables and flourishing weeds. He must keep his garden in order, look after the cultivars and pull out the weeds. Many plants will then find room in his garden and be able to grow, though care is taken that no one plant species gains the upper hand over others. If the defence system is involved in an inflammation of the skin, it will squander its energies there, with the fields in the inner organism left to lie fallow.

Other constitutional problems can also be responsible for a weak digestion, among them anaemia, general exhaustion with a neurasthenic constitution. Poor food quality, for instance vegetables grown in such a way that they are open to fungus attack even in the field, also interferes with intestinal function.

Antibiotics will cut a broad swathe through healthy intestinal flora, and yeasts, for example, then find the ground cleared for them. Cortisone taken by mouth for some time will weaken the whole defence system and this can also affect the intestinal flora.

The best way of detecting yeasts in the intestine is by testing stool samples; a small amount is put in a culture dish. The kind and number of yeasts can then be found by looking at the yeast colonies growing in the culture.

Knowledge that yeasts are forming dense colonies in the intestine indicates to the physician who considers the whole organism of a patient with one of the above four skin conditions that there is a weakness in the digestion. This is the inner aspect of the external skin problem. It needs to be treated as well if one wants to involve the powers of self-healing in the organism's periphery.

Yeasts in the intestine are primarily treated by strengthening the digestion. Medicinal plants containing bitter substances like yellow gentian (*Gentiana lutea*) and chicory (*Cichorium intybus*) act as bitters. Bitter Elixir[2] is recommended (w. sugar, alcohol-free), Gentian[2] (sugar-free, alcohol-free, for people who like it really bitter) and Amara Drops[1] (alcoholic, in a handy small bottle) (S). Antimony in various homoeopathic forms is suitable for treating both intestine and skin (P); Cichorium/Pancreas comp. pilules[2] contain antimony, for instance. Quartz as a homoeopathic medicine regulates the interplay of organ systems, of internal and external organism (P). In some cases the physician will prescribe Digestodoron[1], a medicine for intestinal conditions which contains ferns and a willow extract. Aquilinum comp. pilules[2] work in the same direction.

Something can also be done with diet. Products from biodynamic agriculture may be generally recommended. They are marketed as Demeter produce. Biodynamic farming means that special efforts are made to work with the cosmic qualities that live in light and warmth and have an influence on plants and animals. A wholefood diet rich in roughage is advisable. Avoid industrially refined sugar and white flour, for carbohydrate in this easily assimilated form weakens the powers of digestion (and metabolism in general). Soured milk products and Demeter kvass (traditional Russian drink made from bread) are helpful.

If digestive weakness is so severe that the person concerned does not have the resources to reduce excessive yeast populations to a healthy level, the physician may consider using a drug that kills yeasts. Nystatin is most widely used. It is not taken up into the lining of the intestine and therefore acts only inside the intestine. Follow-up treatment with anthroposophical medicines to prevent relapse is advisable.

Treating skin conditions

Considering the way the skin relates to the whole human being, it is clear that the treatment of skin conditions must often involve the whole organism. Metabolic causes may make it necessary to use medicinal plants to stimulate the function of an organ. Or there may be a general need to stimulate constructive metabolism because the nervous system is too destructive in its functions. This means that internal organ systems often have to be treated as well when dealing with skin conditions.

On the other hand, anthroposophical medical treatment of conditions affecting internal organs may call for external applications to the skin. Bronchitis is greatly relieved by applying mustard packs to the chest; the mustard oils cause mild skin irritation and this draws the inflammatory process away from the bronchi and to the skin. An asthma attack can be cut short with a hot mustard footbath. In this case, the nerves and senses are too active in the lung, causing bronchial muscle spasms; the process is drawn off by stimulating blood flow to the skin at the lower pole of the human form. Just as the skin can be treated via internal organs, so can diseases in the inner organism be treated via the skin.

Here it is interesting to look at nerve connections between internal organs and specific skin areas located directly above these. Reflex arcs that establish a connection to the skin via the spinal marrow can change the volume of blood flow in the fine capillaries of the upper dermis. Where a disposition already exists from other causes, this may in turn help to localize a skin condition in the particular skin area. These reflex connections between skin and internal organs can also be utilized in the treatment of internal organs. Injecting a medicine under the abdominal skin over the liver will have positive effects on the liver simply because of the site chosen for the injection.

We can see from the above that a major part of the treatment must be directed not to the skin itself but elsewhere. It is in the nature of the thing that treatment of the deeper causes, which usually have existed for some time, often for years, cannot be immediately successful. For the length of time needed for this aspect of treatment we can take our orientation from the moon rhythm. The minimum period is usually 28 days, and it will often take several months before the sluggishness of internal organs that has led to skin disorders can be overcome.

Eurythmy and art therapy (painting, drawing, clay-modelling) are an important part of comprehensive anthroposophical treatment. They work in a positive way to enhance the healing process which the physician stimulates with his medicines in the physical body, at levels deep down in the patient's subconscious mind. These therapies start with the patient's conscious efforts to get well. The disease process is thus attacked from two sides, and these approaches complement and strengthen each other. Examples for the frequent use of eurythmy and art therapy are neurodermatitis and melanoma; both will be discussed in more detail in the relevant sections of this book.

Ointments, creams, lotions, compresses and dressings are external applications used in treating skin conditions. They bring fairly quick relief. Homoeopaths have been known to advise against any kind of external treatment, saying that there is a danger of disease processes being displaced from the outside to the inside and then affecting other organ systems. A typical example of such displacement would be asthma developing after highly effective and successful symptomatic external treatment of neurodermatitis. The preconditions for this always exist if the whole organism has not been taken into account and treated as well. We therefore do not believe it to be justifiable to reject the external treatment of skin diseases on principle.

External treatment also eases suffering with skin conditions, though the actual healing process comes with internal treatment. The skin is an organ to which we all have a definite relationship, feeling at one with it. Its treatment with external methods is therefore seen subjectively by patients. This is entirely due to the nature of our skin and cannot be any other way; any treatment of the skin must take this principle into account. Something which helps and benefits one patient may feel unpleasant to another or even aggravate the condition. External applications must therefore be tried out in each individual case. Patients are therefore invited to report their subjective feelings about external treatments; internal treatment is the physician's responsibility.

Considering the fact that substances can be taken in through the skin, one will be careful in choosing the ointment base. Emulsifiers, preservatives, scent, lanolin and so on, both synthetic and of natural origin, can cause sensitization and then allergy. What is more, synthetic ointment ingredients which may not be toxic on their own may nevertheless add their bit to the vast range of environmental influences that are foreign to the body. For the organism must cope with and digest the environmental influences of synthetic products.

Man and nature have been created together and natural substances therefore have a relationship to the human organism and are more easily coped with by the organism than synthetics. It is thanks to the common origin of man and nature that natural substances can have healing properties for human beings. We therefore prefer substances in our medicines for external use that come from the world of nature (animal, vegetable, mineral), just as we do for body care products.

Mineral oils such as vaseline and paraffin come from the inorganic world. They may be said to have no quality at all and thus cannot cause allergies. They keep for unlimited periods and can give the skin a protective fat cover that does not call for any reaction on the part of the organism. An ointment based on vaseline and/or paraffin is exactly right for some very acute inflammatory skin conditions. Ointments containing metals, widely used in anthroposophical medicine, are also based on mineral oils. They stay on the skin surface and are not absorbed, and the metal can develop the required 'radiant' effect directed towards the inner organism.

We would advise against making your own ointments for skin care when there is skin disease. A broad range of body care products made entirely of natural substances is available in pharmacies, drug stores and health food shops, so there is no need to face the risk of variable quality and limited shelf life with home-made ointments.

Treating children's skin

At this point, let us briefly consider why children put up such resistance to anything a physician needs to do in the body boundary, taking blood, for instance, giving an injection or scraping off a molluscum contagiosum. Why are children so afraid of damage being done to the skin?

When an adult says to a child, 'Stop making such a fuss. It can't really hurt,' this shows that he or she does not understand the child's developmental situation. For the child is not yet sure of his body. The sense of touch, the most important sense organ in the skin, allows us to learn as children where our boundaries are. Getting to know those bodily boundaries is a precondition for gaining the right feeling for a boundary in the soul. The adult will then be able to keep the right distance from the outside world. On the other hand the certainty gained in childhood of living in one's own body with its boundaries is also the basis for the adult's certainty in mind and spirit. Certainty then arises that we are sustained and maintained by a divine power. Fear arises when the certainty of being within one's own body, in one's own skin, is lost, and with it also one's trust in God.

In early childhood the relationship to one's physical boundaries, one's own skin, tends to be a loose one. The child, having just come to earth from the spiritual existence he had before birth, has not yet bonded firmly with his body. Because of this, *every* child is afraid of injections, for instance. The 'little prick' of the needle upsets that loose connection between the child's soul and body. This explains why children are afraid of even minor procedures touching the skin. From about the age of ten onwards, bodily awareness, being at home in oneself, is sufficiently secure, so that it is possible to do minor procedures such as scraping off soft warts (molluscum contagiosum) in a calm way, taking time over it.

When children are given anthroposophical medical treatment, it does, however, happen every now and then that injections are necessary. A medicine acts differently if taken by mouth than if it is applied externally or given by injection. For the under-tens, it is a help if their mother provides the missing security in their physical body by keeping loving arms firmly around them. A necessary injection given in an objective, matter-of-course way will never have traumatic consequences.

Special nature of anthroposophical medicines

Most of the medicines used in conventional medicine have been chemically produced. Their effects on physical processes in the organism are compelling, often fast-acting and powerful; yet there are also side-effects. The medicines to which anthroposophical physicians give preference come from the natural world, from the mineral, vegetable or animal worlds. They have been selected on the basis of the inner relationship between man and nature. Both human beings and all other entities in nature have a common evolutionary origin. We are thus able to say that all the processes we observe in minerals, plants and animals can also be found in the complex, many-layered human organism in health and disease. In this sense, the principle established by Paracelsus (1493–1541), which is that the physician must 'pass nature's examination', has been brought to life again in anthroposophical medicine. Thus all possible illnesses human beings may develop lie spread out before us in the plant world; it just needs a trained eye to perceive them.

These medicines are more gentle in their actions, apart from anything else just because nature and man are inwardly related by being subject to the same laws of creation. A medicinal plant may be used undiluted or in a concentrated extract, which is the general method in herbal medicine (phytotherapy). It is also possible to make aqueous or alcoholic solutions and potentize these, that is, dilute step by step, always shaking them rhythmically between stages. This method, originally developed in homoeopathy, is also used with anthroposophical medicines. One part of the original solution (mother tincture) is mixed with nine parts of diluent (diluting medium), shaking rhythmically. This gives us dilution stage (potency) D1 (D stands for 'decimal', i.e. the figure 10, the dilution being in a 1 : 10 ratio). [In the English-speaking world, potencies are given as 1x, 2x, etc., the x standing for the Roman numeral for 10. Tr.] Further 1 : 10 dilution gives us the 2x, etc. The original substance and its properties are gradually left behind and the creative principle which had given rise to the plant emerges. It combines with the diluent and offers a new spectrum of medicinal powers. We call this pharmaceutical process 'potentization'.

The prologue to the Gospel of John starts with these words:

In the beginning was the Word,
and the Word was with God,
and it was a god.
It was with God in the beginning.
All has come into existence through it
and except through the Word
nothing has come about that has arisen.
(based on translation into German by Rudolf Steiner)

This describes how everything material arose from the Word, the divine spirit. In the pharmaceutical process, the spirit is step by step released from the material form it has assumed in the substance.

In conventional medicine, the substance is considered to be the medicine. In the wider concept of anthroposophical pharmacy, special additional treatments add an important quality factor to the medicine. Thus a medicinal plant may be placed in water or alcohol to dissolve out specific substances which are meant to help the human being because they still have vitality. Boiling and distillation bring substances in contact with air, so that used in human beings they create a connection to the soul sphere which has the quality of air. Roasting, reduction to charcoal or to ash subjects substances to intense heat. This gives them a relationship to the human I or self which lives in warmth. In going through a particular pharmaceutical process, the medicinal actions which a substance has are given a specific direction in the human being.

Another special aspect of anthroposophical pharmacy is the use of rhythms from cosmos and earth. The influence that sunlight, coming from the cosmos, has on the earth is different in the morning and in the evening, also due to the influence of always different signs of the zodiac. Water in motion can take in such influences, and because of this, plant extracts must be shaken at specific times in the mornings and evenings. Those cosmic powers are helped to have an influence and enter into the solution by temperature effects. The plant mixture is cooled down to 4°C morning and evening, and heated to 37°C during both day and night. This creates a special medicinal quality. Among other things, the method helps to preserve the medicine.

The use of metals in potentized form is a characteristic aspect of anthroposophical medicine. The human organization is partly con-figured by the powers of the six planets Saturn, Jupiter and Mars on the one hand and Venus, Mercury and Moon on the other, balanced out by the sun which acts as a mediator between these two groups of three. The seven metals which are earthly representatives of those seven planetary influences are shown below, each with one important medicinal action.

Saturn	– lead (Plumbum)	in the 8x, imposes form on excessive vitality
Jupiter	– tin (Stannum)	acts on the relationship between solid and fluid
Mars	– iron (Ferrum)	in the 6x, taking hold of metabolism
Sun	– gold (Aurum)	to strengthen the middle
Mercury	– mercury (Mercurius)	acts on all glands
Venus	– copper (Cuprum)	warming
Moon	– silver (Argentum)	constructive, vitalizing

An alternative to the potentizing of metals is a method used by Weleda where specific medicinal plants are grown in soil treated with the metals. Examples are given below.

Bryophyllum	Argento cultum	– bryophyllum, silver-treated soil
Chelidonium	Ferro cultum	– celandine, iron-treated soil
Cichorium	Stanno cultum	– chicory, tin-treated soil
Hypericum	Auro cultum	– St John's wort, gold-treated soil
Melissa	Cupro culta	– lemon balm, copper-treated soil
Oenothera	Argento culta	– evening primrose, silver-treated soil
Taraxacum	Stanno cultum	– dandelion, tin-treated soil
Urtica dioica	Ferro culta	– stinging nettle, iron-treated soil

Here the metal has been potentized by the plant. A medicinal plant is chosen which shows a relationship to that metal in its vital processes. These 'vegetabilized metals' are particularly helpful when introducing metal therapy, and in metal therapy for children.

Finally there are the 'typical medicines' in anthroposophical medicine. These are compositions of medicinal plants and/or minerals based on our understanding of the threefold nature of the human organism and the four levels of human existence. They will either meet the comprehensive need for healing in an organ system where the potential exists for a number of diseases, or have to do with a specific type of disease (e.g. migraine or hayfever) which often relates closely to our present time and its lifestyle. An example would be Dermatodoron (from the Latin for 'given for the skin'). It contains creeping jenny (*Lysimachia nummularia*) and bittersweet (*Solanum dulcamara*). Creeping jenny can heal wounds and helps the constructive processes, the vitality, of the skin. Bittersweet, a member of the nightshade family, is mildly poisonous and able to limit the excessive metabolism in the skin which may develop in the cold season of the year, for example. It thus has a relationship to the form-giving powers of the human neurosensory system. Dermatodoron is therefore a medicament made with two medical plants that act in polar opposite directions – one addressing the constructive metabolic pole, the other the destructive nerve pole in the skin. The medicinal action arises as the two plants encourage the skin to find the healthy middle way.

Cortisol

Before we come to individual skin conditions and natural methods of treating them, let us consider a medicine widely used in dermatology as a highly effective symptomatic treatment for skin diseases. This is cortisol. It is a vital hormone produced in the adrenal cortex. Its functions are to prepare the organism for stress and reduce inflammation, guiding metabolic processes so that powers of waking consciousness permit rapid action in everyday situations. Cortisol is available in a number of chemical compounds in form of tablets, injections or ointment to reduce inflammation in a wide range of diseases.

With skin conditions, cortisol is best applied externally, as this puts it right on the site of action. With earlier types of cortisol, the anti-inflammatory action always went hand in hand with a suppression of metabolism in the connective tissue cells in the dermis. This meant that the dermis would grow thinner after an extended period of using cortisol; fine blood vessels would stand out, the connective tissue might separate as with stretch marks, and eruptions similar to acne develop.

With the new cortisol compounds used today, the anti-inflammatory action dominates the picture, and the skin-thinning effect is absolutely minimal. Using these new products for a week or two does not cause side-effects. Cortisol to give rapid relief of symptoms with severe allergic contact dermatitis, for instance, where the trigger is an external allergen, or in an acute episode in neurodermatitis, can be seen as a genuine advance in dermatology. It blunts the severity of symptoms and helps to gain time for the slower-acting plant-based and potentized medicines to take effect. Under these conditions, cortisol can have a place also in the approach to medicine broadened through anthroposophy.

Individual skin conditions

Neurodermatitis

We will begin with neurodermatitis, for this is a condition seen most frequently in dermatology. It has become more common in recent decades, and the anthroposophical view of the human being can contribute much to understanding the causes.

The growing incidence of neurodermatitis, especially in children, is characteristic of today's one-sided lifestyle and thinking, and we may indeed call it a disease of our time. Below, we will first consider the kind of skin which is liable to develop neurodermatitis, and then the personal characteristics or soul qualities which may be observed in children and adults. The idea of a threefold organism helps us to see how functions have become one-sided. This makes it possible to establish a diagnosis, and we hope that being able to see through (*dia-gnosis*, Greek for insight based on seeing through things) the external changes in the skin and the psychology, readers will also understand the essential nature of the condition. Once the diagnosis has been made in this sense, it will also point to measures we can take for prevention and treatment.

The term 'atopic' needs to be explained briefly. It refers to reactions that happen in the wrong place (*topos* = Greek for 'place'), and refers to reactions that present as skin inflammation, neurodermatitis; the term 'atopic dermatitis' is also used. Reactions in the mucous membranes of the respiratory tract and eyes include hay fever (allergic rhinitis), allergic conjunctivitis and asthma. Space being limited, only hay fever will be considered in this book, since dermatologists, also being trained in allergology, often treat this as well.

Tendency to develop neurodermatitis

Apart from people who have neurodermatitis we also know others who have a particular type of skin and a tendency to develop neuro-dermatitis even though their skin is healthy. This is evident from specific signs in the skin that are referred to as 'signs of an atopic skin diathesis'. It means a tendency to develop neurodermatitis of the skin, and hay fever and asthma on the mucous membranes. The skin signs relating to this are described on the next page.

Skin with a tendency to neurodermatitis is dry. It looks sallow and dull, sometimes grey, its surface saltlike because of fine skin flakes. The dryness is due to a reduction in specific fats in the spaces between cornified cells in the upper epidermis (see the section on the epidermis, pages 6ff). As a result, water is lost to the outside from the epidermis. Water is also less well retained in the epidermis because of a lack of urea. The sebaceous glands produce less sebum and the sweat glands less sweat. These symptoms suggest a loss of constructive powers in the skin.

People with a tendency to develop neurodermatitis sweat less than others. If they do some heavy work and get into a sweat after all, the skin will itch for a time. Baths and showers dry out the skin more quickly, so that it is liable to feel tight and itchy afterwards. Sheep's wool often cannot be tolerated close to the skin; it can cause itching and even dermatitis. Wool fibres are relatively thick and very curly; they can therefore give the skin a 'micro-massage'. The skin with its careful balance between nerve and blood reacts to this by slightly increasing blood flow and this makes it warm. The skin of people with a tendency to develop neurodermatitis will however react one-sidedly in the nerves, that is, with itching.

The most interesting and telling sign is 'white dermographia', meaning the possibility of producing white writing on the skin. Moving a blunt fingernail across the skin on the stomach, using light pressure, causes normal skin to respond soon after by producing a red line, a sign that blood flow has increased. People tending to develop neurodermatitis will, however, produce a white line; the 'coat of nerves' is overreacting. Nerves supplying the musculature of blood vessels in the skin cause the muscle fibres to contract; the vessels narrow, and a narrow line on either side of the line made by the nail has less blood supplied to it. This causes the skin to turn white.

Imbalance in the relation between blood and nerve is also evident in the hands and feet. Reduced circulation makes them cold and sometimes a bit blue. Increased sensitivity of the visual nerve, the biggest nerve in the head, shows itself in an inability to tolerate bright sunlight. This gives us a whole number of phenomena which characterize people who tend to get neurodermatitis as having a skin where nerves are hyperactive, 'nervy'; skin that is 'charged', as it were. The skin is wide awake and tends to be excessively awake.

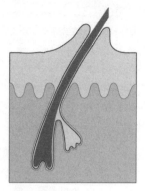

Cone of horn on a hair
(keratosis pilaris)

Form-giving powers also attack with more vigour, drawing lines in the skin. Examples are increased numbers of wrinkles in the lips and palms. One or two deep folds may be found even in the lids of infants with atopic skin diathesis, pulling the lower lid away from the inner angle of the eye.

Another constitutional sign is keratosis pilaris, with increased cornification at the points where hairs emerge from the skin. Small cornified cones develop that make the skin feel like a cheese grater. They appear mainly on the sides of the upper arms and thighs, less often on the cheeks. The cones may stand out more from the reddened skin and are particularly disliked by girls in early puberty who are concerned about their appearance.

People with a tendency to develop neurodermatitis often have dark shadows (haloes) under their eyes. It makes them look as if they'd never got enough sleep, though this is not necessarily the case. They tend to be tall, slender or thin, the asthenic constitutional type. One often sees two whorls of hair on the head – one on the back of the head and another to the right just above the forehead.

An allergy to nickel is often seen; it is not statistically proven but known from experience in dermatological practice. It is usually acquired in childhood from the use of ear studs containing nickel, and affected mainly women until some years ago. Now that fashion makes men also wear them, the allergy is quite often seen in men.

A second common form of intolerance exists with regard to some foods – cow's milk, citrus fruit, strawberries and tomatoes. The causes of such intolerances in the organism as a whole will be considered later. With cow's milk, people may simply have an aversion, or it causes digestive problems such as sensation of fullness, wind, diarrhoea or constipation. Taking cow's milk can also aggravate existing neurodermatitis. Citrus fruit, strawberries and tomatoes may do the same, or also produce small spots on the skin that will persist for some days. Strawberries can also trigger nettle rash. Other, less common food intolerances will be considered later.

In people tending to develop neurodermatitis, and even more so in those who have the condition, the organism's defence system shows an imbalance between the resistance provided by immunoglobulins, which are proteins in the blood, and resistance through specialized cells (antibodies). One of the immunoglobulins, immunoglobulin E (IgE) is often present at high levels in the blood. This increased readiness to react to foreign substances can cause allergic asthma or hay fever. With both conditions, the allergic reaction is located in the mucous membranes. Elevated IgE levels can also affect the skin. The immunoglobulin can migrate from the blood to the epidermis and attach itself to the defence cells there. If the individual is already sensitized to dust mites, for instance, an existing neurodermatitis will get worse when much dust is raised when doing housework.

On the one hand, the tendency to react to the environment with defensive proteins is excessive, on the other hand, cell-based defence reactions are often poorly developed in people with atopic skin diathesis. This weakness makes the skin susceptible to infection – warts (ordinary and molluscum contagiosum), herpes, impetigo and fungal infection are seen in children, especially those with dry skin. This does not mean, of course, that the defences of the whole organism are weakened as is the case with HIV infection and the serious condition known as AIDS. Only the part of the immune system connected with the skin is affected.

Personality traits of adults with neurodermatitis

It is often intelligent people who tend to develop neurodermatitis. Their neurosensory system has been wide awake from birth, and so they have taken in much of the world around them. This has helped their powers of observation and thought from the beginning – constitutionally so, as it were. This kind of intelligence does, however, quite often tend to be somewhat one-sided. The emphasis is on the head, the intellect, tending to be very much of this world, and one-sidedly reacting rapidly to sensory perceptions. Yet their own bodies are often felt to be something foreign. An inner life where the emphasis is on the head can lead to brooding too much about oneself and strict self-control. Always ready to take action, at work for instance, they tend to ignore tiredness and the fact that they've taken on too much. They do not realize they are doing too much, and soldier on in spite of growing exhaustion. The soul is then not able to come free of the body for night-time rest and a form of sleeping disorder develops. This also explains why these patients often suffer from pruritus when undressing at night and on going to sleep. The soul has got caught up in the skin and is unable to relax into sleep in that intermediate stage between day and night.

Too much activity in the senses means that professionally they like to work with computers and to sit in front of the television when at home. Being so wide awake, they are predestined to work in data processing. Their superiors value the work they do and encourage them further. Computers are, however, an extension of brain-bound thinking placed in the machine's network of electronic links. Working on computers can therefore increase the one-sidedness in an overactive neurosensory system. A liking for television proves equally harmful, a kind of inverted 'similia similibus' (treat like with like), and leads to illness. It is interesting to note that people who spend a lot of time in front of a screen are insensitive to potentized medicines and more difficult to treat.

Personality traits of children with neurodermatitis

In conclusion we describe the impression a physician gains when a child tending to develop neurodermatitis comes to the consulting room. A young patient, two years old, looks wide-eyed at the physician. After a minute this new person in a white coat is no longer of interest and he climbs down from his mother's lap. Looking around the consulting room he is fascinated by the light switches and the shelf with many tubes of ointments. These are the early signs of an interest in technology and electrical appliances, and also in things that are differentiated, set out in organized arrays (shelf of ointments). He does not stay with anything for long, moving on from one impression to another. Motor activity is quite often considerable, even to the point of restlessness. From there it is not far to the fidgeter with hyperkinetic syndrome.

Minor forms of neurodermatitis

In most cases, neurodermatitis persists for a limited time and symptoms are not severe. Milk crust (cradle cap) may appear a few weeks after birth, yellow scaling, sometimes thick and usually firmly adherent on the scalp. The name 'milk crust' does not refer to milk being the cause but to the appearance of the lesion which looks rather like the dried-up skin on hot milk. The skin is reddened, and the redness may also appear on the face, forehead and sides of cheeks.

The corners of the mouth may show redness of inflammation with a horizontal fissure; these are also called perleches.

In winter, dryness can cause the lips to crack and become inflamed; the whole area around the mouth may also be reddened, with dry scales.

The fold between ear lobe and cheek may be inflamed and show cracks.

Winter is always a critical time for people with a tendency to develop neurodermatitis. Toe pads may grow more cornified and develop cracks that may be painful. This is the 'atopic winter foot'.

Children with dry skin will sometimes have grey scales at the back of the neck that do not wash off. This is due to low-grade chronic skin inflammation. Mild inflammation not recognizable as such is also the cause of coin-sized, not clearly defined foci with fine scales and reduced pigmentation, usually on the cheeks.

Dermatitis on the nipples of nursing mothers is a mild form of neurodermatitis. Nursing infants clearly stress the nipples if these cannot recover adequately between feeds.

The appearance of fully developed neurodermatitis in different age groups

The skin changes seen with neurodermatitis are called eruptions, indicating that a disease process is affecting the skin from the inside and going to the outside. The medical term is eczema or dermatitis, which simply means inflammation of the skin. The causes of dermatitis may lie in the organism (e.g. triggered by nerves) or outside (e.g. cleaning materials). In either case, it looks the same and follows the same laws.

Initially the skin grows red and swollen. Small nodules then develop that may turn into vesicles. If the inflammation is severe, the vesicles merge into weeping areas that soon dry out and form crusts. If the inflammation calms down, the skin goes through a stage where it grows scaly. Slight redness will persist for some weeks to remind one of the healed dermatitis. At all stages, pruritus (itching) may be more or less severe. It is the most unpleasant part of neurodermatitis, may be worse at night and make it difficult to sleep for all age groups. Lack of sleep and exhausted nerves will in turn make the pruritus worse again.

The dermatitis may appear soon after birth. It usually starts with milk crust on the scalp and spreads to the whole face (except for the region around the mouth), the throat and back of the neck. Later the backs of the hands and wrists may be affected as well. In the nappy region, the skin can get inflamed as conditions are like those in a humid chamber. It can also happen, however, that neurodermatitis affects all skin areas except for the nappy region. In infants and young children the dermatitis tends to be weeping.

Between the ages of three and seven, the extensor surfaces or sides of limbs are mainly affected. But dermatitis may also develop on the inside of the elbow and back of the knee. They tend to attract bacteria (staphylococci and streptococci) and have moist crusts. The lymph nodes connected with the affected skin area can usually be felt to be enlarged and are sensitive to pressure (axillae [armpits] and groin, under the lower jaw, at the back of the neck). In very general terms we can say that dermatitis at the back of the knee is more likely to have its causes in the metabolic sphere (e.g. digestive weakness), dermatitis on the inside of the elbow in the typical 'excessive nerviness' of the skin. 'Sandbox dermatitis' develops when children play in damp sand out of doors in the spring; air and moisture dry out the skin on the back of the hand and the forearms, and this causes the dermatitis.

Between seven and 21 years of age is the real time for flexure (bend) dermatitis. The tendency is now to dryness, to skin thickening with severe itching. Very itchy, solid small nodules may also develop at this age and persist for months. Hay fever and asthma may develop as well.

In adulthood, neurodermatitis is generally localized in the upper pole of the body – head, neck, low-neckline area, shoulders, upper part of the back and hands. This shows the relationship of the condition to the neurosensory system. It is often triggered by nerve strain and overwork, during exam times or through conflicts with partners. The eruption tends to appear not during the actual time of stress but quite often only afterwards, when the stress is getting less and the individual relaxes. As nerves get less stressed, the powers of the blood take the stage, creating new imbalances and making the skin bloom into eruption.

Causes of neurodermatitis

People tending to develop neurodermatitis show one-sided situations and imbalances in the skin, with reduced vitality, increased imposition of form and more nerve activity. The skin is too much awake, too 'nervy'. The individual's soul and spirit is too active in the whole neurosensory system and especially also in the skin. The older term 'neurodermatitis' is therefore appropriate. Other, more recent terms such as 'endogenous dermatitis (endogenous = to come from inside) and 'atopic dermatitis' point to less important characteristics of this skin condition. One-sided involvement of the human soul and I in the neurosensory system means that they are less active in other areas in the organism, above all in the digestion.

A weak digestion and reduced anabolism (building up, constructive function) and also a weak constitution are the inner aspect of the external skin problem. Weak digestion does not mean constipation, but stomach, liver, gall bladder, pancreas and intestines being less able to break down foods with the help of digestive juices. The aim of digestive function must be to reduce the foods to their building blocks and remove the foreign nature of the life form from which they have come. Only then should they pass through the intestinal wall into the blood. In someone with neurodermatitis whose digestion is weak, the substances taken into the blood still have a bit of that foreign nature when they reach the blood. Foreign matter in the blood is poison, however, and must be eliminated. Elimination does happen then, but via the skin. This is not designed to cope with the situation to such a degree, however, and becomes inflamed. Here we have the causes of food intolerance and indeed allergies. Excessive nerve activity may thus be joined by a weak digestion as a cause of neurodermatitis.

The fact that soul and I are less focused on metabolism also has another consequence with neurodermatitis. The I is less connected with the warmth organism and therefore also with fat metabolism, which is the physical basis on which body warmth develops. This explains the three characteristics of someone who merely tends to develop neurodermatitis but has not yet got it:

- the epidermis is dry because fat lamellae between horn cells have been reduced;
- the lower dermis produces less fat in its sebaceous glands;
- the dermis contains less fatty tissue, so that the person is of slender build.

Using the anthroposophical view of the human being to help us understand the body language of someone with that tendency, we know how we can meet the needs of such people as regards prevention and treatment.

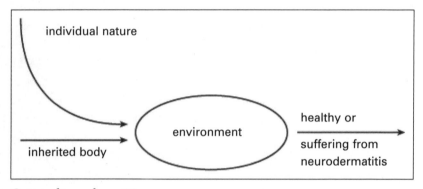

Causes of neurodermatitis

The human I connects progressively with its physical body during embryonic development, birth and also after this. Prior to conception, this I existed only in the spirit. The individual is born into a particular environment in his living body. Causes for neurodermatitis come from three directions – what the individual has brought with him, the body inherited from his parents, and the environment.

Listening to people with neurodermatitis who were born in the 1990s, the impression is that the I finds it more and more difficult to resist the attractions of the sense-perceptible world. These young people are easily absorbed into the world around them through their sense organs. This would be one reason why the neurosensory process is too active.

Another reason is that these young people are less and less able to overcome inherited tendencies for disease. After birth, the inherited body is mainly individualized through febrile infectious conditions such as the classic childhood diseases and febrile inflammations of the upper respiratory tract. Up to eight febrile colds a year are normal in young children. Metaphorically speaking the inherited body is recast in the right form in the fire of the fever, 'sweating out' any tendency to develop neurodermatitis.

The environment into which a child with that tendency is born presents many things to him today that are liable to transform the tendency into manifest disease:

- a flood of sensory stimuli
- lack of rhythm in everyday life
- pollution of air, water and foods.

The many sensory stimuli are attractive to young children today and the spiritual world from which they have come to earth is all too soon forgotten. As a result, the children lack protection in soul and spirit. Parents are challenged to become aware of our spiritual nature as human beings so that they can truly create the protective mantle which only parents can provide for their child.

Prevention

It is not uncommon to see neurodermatitic eruptions heal up when a child has overcome a febrile infection. It is therefore advisable to avoid fever-reducing medicines and antibiotics wherever possible. Febrile infections can usually be well managed with the methods known in natural medicine, and there need be no complications. Childhood diseases should not all be made impossible with comprehensive vaccination programmes. Very generally speaking, only vaccination against polio, tetanus and diphtheria can be recommended; all others should at least be given careful thought. It is now known that frequent febrile infections in childhood reduce the frequency of allergies and cancer in adulthood. This has been demonstrated in a study published in the *Lancet* in May 1999. A total of 675 Swedish school children were compared, half of them from Waldorf Steiner schools, the others from conventional schools in the same local area as the Waldorf Steiner school. It was found that Waldorf pupils, especially those with an 'anthroposophical lifestyle', had distinctly fewer allergies than the pupils in the other group. 'Anthroposophical lifestyle' was the term used for a way of life which meant the following for the boys and girls in question:

- they were given far fewer antibiotics and fever-reducing medicines, fewer vaccinations;
- they had had more infectious diseases such as measles, German measles and chickenpox, and
- eaten a more ecological diet, especially lactic-acid fermented vegetables.

The study showed that changing our western lifestyle can reduce the incidence of neurodermatitis by half. We simply must allow children to have the classic childhood diseases and cut down on the use of anti-biotics and fever-reducing medicines.

How can parents create that protective mantle for a child with neurodermatitis? They must first of all ask themselves if they truly accept the child who has come to them as he is, including his skin problems. Anything which is other than expected, difficult character traits such as the defiance and obstinacy that get on one's nerves, must be loved just as much as the positive sides which one is happy to accept. Grace at meals, bed-time prayers, good-night songs and stories feed the child's mind and spirit. Fairy tales offer a world of images that reflect the spiritual situation of human beings, and children have no difficulty in understanding their language. The rhythm of the festivals of the seasons gives a sequence of events that are always returning and relate to things of the spirit by which the child can feel himself to be sustained and supported deep down and unconsciously.

The fostering of religion of a kind that is right for a child offers both prevention and treatment, for religion (from the Latin *religere* = reconnect) connects human beings who are in physical existence with their spiritual reality, their divine origin.

Television sets, radios and electronic toys are not suitable for children. The sensory stimuli coming from them do nothing but destroy vitality, not adding to it in any way. The tendency to develop neuro-dermatitis is increased when children use electronic appliances. This does, of course, also apply to adults when such use goes beyond a certain measure, as with television, for instance.

Other sensory stimuli help the healthy development of the sense organs and hence also the child's whole physical body. Unvarnished blocks made of different kinds of wood help to train the sense of touch – the wood of fir, beech or oak has a different colour, weight, firmness, surface and grain. A plastic brick does not offer all these sensory qualities and opportunities for discovery. Simple wooden blocks also offer other advantages over Lego bricks. They offer more possibility to have variation and stimulate the imagination. Preformed plastic bricks are simply connected with each other and will stay together. With wooden blocks, on the other hand, you learn about statics, about above and below, gravity and buoyancy. It is important, therefore, to consider the quality of playthings.

The abilities of children with a tendency to develop neurodermatitis tend to be one-sided and it is therefore necessary to help their powers of imagination. Wide awake, they are well able to take things in and react quickly, sometimes too much so. To balance this out, one needs to encourage them to become involved in the arts — painting, modelling, craft work, singing and playing instruments. Waldorf Steiner education provides exactly this, pure prevention if there are tendencies to develop neurodermatitis.

Breast-feeding is another form of prevention. If one parent or even both parents have hay fever, asthma, neurodermatitis or even just a very dry skin, it is advisable to breast-feed for a full six months. More than six months means that the gradual process of separation from the mother, the 'birth' into independent feeding, is delayed too much, which may sometimes result in delays in psychological development. Mothers should base their diet on sour-milk products rather than fresh cow's milk whilst breast-feeding and cut down on eggs, fish and wheat flour. This avoids the danger of their digestion being weakened and proteins appearing in breast milk that demand too much of the infant at this stage. It is also best to avoid citrus fruit, refined sugar, sweets, animal fats (lard, dripping, fatty meat) and hot spices.

Treatment

External applications will at the least provide relief. Dry skin conditions call for ointments with a fat basis. Occasionally, fat-based ointments are also not tolerated, for the fat creates an occlusive film on the skin surface, with the inflammation underneath and the irritation getting worse. In that case one needs moisturizing creams that let air pass through. Red, itching and indeed weeping dermatitic lesions can be soothed with products containing zinc oxide applied at night (S).

As already stated, treatment for the skin must be individual. The same ointment can benefit one person and have no effect or even prove harmful for another. A number of suggestions will therefore be made for external treatment. The decision as to which to use has to be based on trial and error.

Fat-based ointments (S):
- SK ointment base[1], special manufacture with 10% of sea buckthorn seed oil [not available in the UK, Tr.]
- Rosatum Heilsalbe (wound-healing ointment)[2]
- Hametum Ointment made with witch hazel (*Hamamelis virginiana*) extract by Schwabe
- Dermatodoron Ointment[1], esp. for very dry skin of children; contains bittersweet (*Solanum dulcamara*) and creeping jenny (*Lysimachia nummularia*)
- Mercurialis comp. Ointment[2], with extract of dog's mercury (*Mercurialis perennis*)
- Birch Cream with beeswax as an antibacterial

Non-greasy creams, easily absorbed into the skin:
- Dr Hauschka Hand Cream with extract of bryophyllum, also suitable for general body care
- Almond Intensive Facial Cream[1], a composition free from any kind of irritant; can be mixed with Almond Facial Oil[1] to increase the fat content to meet individual needs
- Birch Cream natural – antibacterial
- Horsetail tea 50% in an ointment base; contains 50% of water. It is best to ask a pharmacist to make this up; the formula is:

Equisetum arvense, Decoctum aquosum 10%   50.0
(freshly made)
Ungt. emulsificans   ad 100.0
M. f. ungt.

Alternatively, Eucerin anhydrous may be used for the ointment base (contains wool alcohols). These creams with high water content do not contain preservatives and must be stored in a refrigerator to prevent their going mouldy.

Products containing zinc oxide:
- Calendula Moisturizing Baby Cream[1]
- Hypericum 25% oil[2], 10% in soft zinc paste (pasta zinci mollis)

- Mirfulan (ointment manuf. by Merckle), contains 10% of cod-liver oil

During acute episodes with extensive inflammatory redness and a tendency for lesions to weep it is helpful to apply compresses providing fat and moisture. First apply a cream (e.g. the horsetail cream above) to affected skin areas; this prevents the moist compress from extracting too much fat from the skin. For the compress itself use heartsease tea (*Viola tricolor*), for example. If a whole limb or perhaps the trunk needs to be treated, use tubular bandages such as Tubifast (viscose and elastane) of suitable size.

Oil dispersion baths do more than supply the skin with fats. The special apparatus (Jungebad, Bad Boll, Germany) disperses a medicated oil (olive oil with herbal extracts) so finely in the water that extremely small droplets of it are distributed throughout the water. The oil then reaches deeper levels in the skin, stimulating the warmth organism in general and calling up powers of self-healing. Dispersion bath oils[2] with horsetail extract (Equisetum ex herba W 5%, Oleum) and Rose Oil (Rosae floribus 10%, Oleum) are best for people with neurodermatitis (S). Warmth is also stimulated by just applying pure oil to the whole body at night (healthy as well as affected skin); Malva comp. Oil[2] or Lavender 10% Oil[2] are suitable for this (S). Intolerance is rare with natural essential oils.

Internal treatment using medicines based on animal, vegetable and mineral substances is designed to support anabolism, building up substances, in the whole organism and especially the skin to counteract excessive destructive actions on the part of the neurosensory system. Potentized silver (Argentum) (P) serves this purpose, for example. Very small doses of quartz (P) can help to correct the balance between internal organs and skin. Weakened powers of digestion can be stimulated using medicinal plants that contain bitter principles, an example being yellow gentian (*Gentiana lutea*) (P). Children who do not tolerate cow's milk and tend to have recurrent tonsillitis, nasal polyps and middle-ear inflammation need calcium in homoeopathic doses (P).

Self-medication to treat neurodermatitis internally:
- to stimulate digestive powers:
  Bitter Elixir[2] (with sugar, alcohol-free)

Gentian Stomach Tonic[2] (no sugar and alcohol-free)
Gentiana comp. Globuli[2] (pilules), esp. for young children
Amara Drops[1] (alcoholic)

- to stimulate elimination via the kidneys:
Nierentonikum[2] (kidney tonic)
- to calm the nerves and for sleeping problems:
Passiflora Nerventonikum[2] (nerve tonic)
Passiflora Zaepfchen and Kinderzaepfchen[2] (suppositories and paediatric suppositories)
- for wet, acute inflammation and dermatitis behind the ears and at the back of the knees, for dermatitis where the emphasis is on metabolism:
Dulcamara/Lysimachia Drops[1], 5–10 drops three times daily before meals for children, 10–30 drops three times daily before meals for adults.
The drops can increase the itching with dry, itching dermatitis (emphasis on nerves) and are not suitable in this case.

Seed oils with specific unsaturated fatty oils, especially gamma linolenic acid, are somewhere between being medicines and food supplements. Evening primrose and borage oil contain these beneficial fatty acids; we prefer the first and recommend the form that is not in capsules. It can be bought in pharmacies (Oleum oenothera) who obtain it wholesale. One teaspoonful/day for children, two teaspoons/day for adults (S). Buy only 100 ml of fresh oil at a time and store in a cool, dark place. In that way you can be sure it will not spoil. The unsaturated fatty acids help to develop the fat lamellae between horn cells in the epidermis and reduce the tendency to hypersensitivity reactions in the body boundaries. The effect is more marked in children than in adults.

Eurythmy therapy can be a great help. It was developed by Rudolf Steiner and plays an important role in anthroposophical medicine. Eurythmy therapy is a movement therapy where the spoken word is not produced by the organs of speech but allowed to pass through the whole human form. There is a specific movement of arms, legs and trunk relating to every speech sound. The gesture acts inwards and into the sphere of the internal organs. Exercises may be given, for example, to compensate for a tendency for sense organs to be hypersensitive; used regularly for some time they give the individual a 'thicker skin'. Trained eurythmy therapists work in collaboration with a physician. Young children will do the exercises together with their mothers (or fathers).

Art therapy can also be a help with neurodermatitis. Painting therapy serves to exercise the soul's ability to go along with perceptions of colour. Sensory perceptions and the inner response to them, which tend to go apart in people suffering from neurodermatitis, are brought together again.

Sea climate and mountain air help people with neurodermatitis to gain a healthy, stable skin. Sea air makes you tired and hungry, stimulating metabolic functions. A period in the mountains has a slightly different effect. The organism is subtly 'nourished' via the senses and thus is given fresh impulses by impressions gained in the world of nature. Metabolism is thus both stimulated and given form.

Let us briefly consider the treatment of the milder forms of neurodermatitis. Horsetail baths are recommended for the milk crust of infants and young children (S). Once a week add a tea to the bathwater, which is made by putting a handful of dried horsetail into about a litre of boiling water, letting it boil for 5 minutes and then draw for another 15 minutes, then strain and add to the bathwater. After the bath, apply Calendula Baby Oil[1] or Dr Hauschka Rose Body Moisturizer to the scalp and leave to act for 10 minutes. Finally use a soft brush to remove the scales and crust.

Keratosis pilaris is a constitutional sign of atopic skin diathesis. If one does not want to wait until it gradually disappears of its own accord after puberty, it helps (temporarily) to soften the cornified cones by soaking in a full bath or taking a sauna and then towelling briskly. Body care to moisturize the skin will make the skin changes less obvious (S).

Dermatitis of the nipples when breast-feeding is helped by applying Calendula Cream[1] to the areola, and Hypericum/Calendula Ointment[1] directly to the nipples, especially if cracks (rhagades) have formed (S). Mundbalsam (oral balm)[2] is also helpful here. Cracks in the nipple can attract bacteria and this may lead to mastitis. To prevent cracks, the mother-to-be can wash her breasts daily with sage tea during pregnancy; this has a mild tannin effect (S). Dr Hauschka Lemon Body Oil also helps to prevent cracks.

Perleches and rhagades at the ear heal if Calendula Baby Cream[1] is applied at night and Hypericum/Calendula Ointment[1] during the day (S). This ointment can be used to deal with any kind of rhagades on hands and feet, applying it lavishly and covering with a plaster (S).

The description of skin with a tendency to develop neurodermatitis clearly showed that textiles can also be a problem. Apart from sheep's wool, synthetic fabrics tend to be a problem as they hold in moisture and body heat. Cotton is best tolerated and generally also silk. Makers' labels made of synthetic fabric are best removed from clothes as they irritate the skin. Allergic skin reactions to textile dyes may also develop. Materials dyed blue or black contain the most dye; cheap synthetics often do not hold the dye well so that sweat will dissolve it out. If it seems likely that a dermatitis has been caused by clothing, undyed cotton would be the best choice.

Dietary problems and advice

The 'inner aspect' of neurodermatitis is the digestive weakness we have been discussing; it causes food intolerances of all kinds and also genuine allergies. Intolerance and allergy may be evident in the intestines themselves in the form of constipation, diarrhoea, wind, sensation of fullness or abdominal pain. Or patient and physician get a warning when the skin condition worsens, usually within half a day of taking the food concerned. A particular food that is suspected of aggravating the neurodermatitis or causes intestinal problems should be avoided for two to four weeks. After this, eat a good quantity of it to provoke a reaction. This is the most reliable way of testing foods for intolerance. The table on the next page lists foods that are good and not good for people with neurodermatitis. This is based on the most common intolerances and also on general value for a healthy diet.

People with neurodermatitis serve as indicators for the quality of environmental conditions; this holds true especially for foods. Environmental pollution, over-breeding, genetic modification, overuse of fertilizers, plant protectives, veterinary medicines, and a high degree of industrial processing have a negative influence on foods. Three examples may serve to demonstrate the danger which threatens the quality of foods today – wheat, carrots and cow's milk. In recent decades, following the Second World War, wheat went through major

Good	Not good
millet*, buckwheat*	in some cases wheat, rye
	refined sugar
spelt, barley	sweets, white flour
wholegrains	
honey, maple syrup	
green salads, beetroot	fish and egg in large quantities
carrots, broccoli, courgettes,	
[Swiss] chard,	
organically grown vegetables	
butter**	whole milk, soya products
sour milk products	pork, offal
vegetable oils	
sea buckthorn juice (vitamin C)	citrus fruit, kiwi, strawberries,
almonds, pears, mild apples	sour fruit, tomatoes, sweet peppers,
	multivitamin juices, hot spices,
	ketchup, alcohol,
	synthetic colouring, preservatives
	and aromas

* Place in boiling water, pour water off and cook in fresh water.
** Butter is usually well tolerated.

Eat with caution

peanuts, hazelnuts, walnuts
hard cheeses, animal fats
peppers, radish, chives,
celeriac/celery

changes produced by breeding. Varieties were adapted to the large amounts of mineral nitrogenous fertilizer used in conventional agriculture, and the protein (gluten) was hardened to serve baking technology (high volume) by increasing the proportion of certain proteins with low sulphur content. This means that wheat protein now contains less sulphur. Sulphur is, however, the bearer of qualities of light and warmth. Too much low-sulphur gluten therefore makes wheat less tolerable. For people with neurodermatitis it is advisable to use spelt, a grain which will also grow on poor soils and (depending on the variety) has not been changed to the same extent by breeding.

It has been the custom for generations to give puréed carrots to infants when weaning. Carrot is a food of high quality and has always been well tolerated. The red pigment, provitamin A (carotene) is important for visual function in the fundus of the eye, a sign that carrot is of special value in building up the whole neurosensory system, including the skin. It makes carrot an actual medicine for someone with neurodermatitis, when the anabolic aspect has suffered in the skin. However, for about ten years now, parents have reported when bringing their children to see the dermatologist that carrot causes the children to develop skin eruptions. Observations have been made which suggest that hybridization of carrot seed is responsible for this. Techniques to change seed using mechanical, chemical, electrical and radioactive manipulation are used in laboratories. This explains a loss of quality which even biodynamic growing methods cannot balance out. It is therefore recommended to eat carrots grown from non-hybridized seed. Ask for such carrots in your health-food store or get such seed and grow your own.

Cattle have been the most important domesticated animals for millennia. Cow's milk and products based on it are an important part of truly human nutrition. When a child with neurodermatitis does not tolerate cow's milk well, we have to consider how this milk is produced. It is wrong to speak of this milk simply as 'protein from another species'. Cow's milk from biodynamic farms — where the cow still has its horns, goes out to pasture and is fed hay — is often better tolerated than milk from conventionally run farms. Processing whole milk using lactic-acid producing bacteria to obtain sour milk products (buttermilk, kefir, *filmjölk* [Swedish-style soured milk, Tr.], yoghurt, quark) makes it more digestible. The work the bacteria do to break down milk protein is a kind of predigestion, relieving people with weak digestions of some of the work.

When you have found a food which intestines and skin, or both, cannot cope with in yourself or a child, it is advisable to try it again after some time. It is certainly possible that the organism's readiness to break out into dermatitis has settled down in the meantime and the allergic tendency has disappeared. You must not, of course, run risks with a severe allergy that has been formally established (to peanuts, for instance). On the other hand it would be wrong to limit the range of foods you are able to eat more and more, depriving the organism of the opportunity to come to terms with a food once the weakness has been overcome.

It has already been suggested that infants should be breast-fed for six months. If the child has extensive neurodermatitis, the mother should avoid fresh whole milk and take soured milk products instead. If this does not lead to improvement, omit all milk products for four weeks and see if the dermatitis improves. The nursing mother will get the calcium she needs from almonds, goat's and sheep's cheeses, green cabbage varieties and pulses. After the six months, begin to wean the infant by slowly introducing other foods. Almond milk is recommended for this:

Almond milk
125 g finely ground peeled almonds
1000 g strained oat or rice gruel (made with about 50 g of oats or rice)
50 g lactose (from health food store)

It is also possible to give goat's or mare's milk if available. Mare's milk is the more valuable of the two; it is, however, expensive to obtain. Giving almond milk on its own will provide the child with sufficient calcium but not the vitamin B_{12} required. Because of this, almond milk should always be combined with genuine milk.

Infants and young children with neurodermatitis should never be given raw cereals soaked in water. This would ask too much of their powers of digestion; fresh grain may also cause allergies to develop more quickly. The use of heat in preparing cereals, soaking the grain or meal, heating it and letting it swell to its full extent, makes them digestible for the children. Ready-made baby foods of Demeter quality are available and very suitable (e.g. Holle brand).

Psoriasis (psoriasis vulgaris)

This condition is the polar opposite of neurodermatitis. It is also one of the most common skin conditions.

Signs and symptoms

Under the microscope, a skin sample from a psoriatic lesion shows greatly elongated papillae in the upper dermis, and these contain extended, serpentine capillaries filled with blood to the limit. Blood serum seeps from the capillaries, and many inflammatory cells are found near them which may also migrate to the epidermis and collect in tiny lakes of pus. In these psoriatic lesions, the blood therefore moves centrifugally with excessive might from body interior to periphery beneath the epidermis. The impression is that this imposes excessive metabolism on the epidermis. It thickens, horn cells mature too soon and incompletely. The migration of a horn cell from the lowest level of the epidermis to the surface takes not the normal 28 but only 3 or 4 days. Increased amounts of fat are deposited between horn cells. Precipitate cell maturation in the epidermis of psoriasis lesions explains why the skin is so scaly.

The lesions have three characteristics. The thick scales, sometimes plaquelike, can be scraped off like candle grease. If you continue to scrape you come to a final thin membrane. Take this away as well and drops of blood appear like dew, due to the fact that the tips of the papillae in the upper dermis with their blood-filled capillaries have been opened up.

The most common psoriatic lesion is a sharply defined, often thickened red plaque in the front part of the knees and on the elbows. (This is exactly the opposite position to the eruption seen with neurodermatitis which develops on the other side of the joint.) Other frequently affected areas are the hairy scalp, buttocks, genital region and nails. If the condition has spread more, lesions also appear over the lower back (sacrum). Trunk and extremities may show numerous

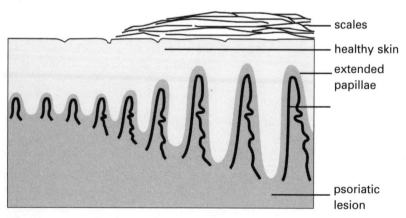

Skin specimen with psoriatic lesion seen under the microscope

palm-sized lesions that may also merge to cover larger areas. Finally it can also happen that the whole body is affected, with no area left free.

Psoriasis mostly develops first in childhood or youth. It will then disappear, only to come up again on specific occasions. Very rarely it may first appear after the age of 50 or even later. An acute form mostly occurs in childhood as an eruption in small spots all over the body. It is triggered by infections such as suppurative tonsillitis. On the other hand the condition may be extremely chronic, persisting for decades, with the lesions always in the same sites (e.g. knees, elbows, lower back). The skin lesions are generally better in summer, but regularly get worse in winter.

People suffering from psoriasis do not infrequently also show irregularities in metabolism – uric acid, blood fats and blood sugar may be elevated and even need treatment. Psoriasis may also affect the joints, causing painful inflammation. The typical person with neurodermatitis tends to be tall and thin; someone with psoriasis will often be sturdily built and tend to put on weight.

Reflecting on the personal traits of people with psoriasis, an above-average number of them are able to cope with mental stress, tolerant and sociable, and not too fussy about things in everyday life. They like the occasional drink, for instance, though they know that this may make the psoriasis worse. They are not always reliable when it comes to taking medicines. Many are highly active people and inwardly impatient. They'd like to get as much as possible done in a short time. This means that they are often highly successful in their occupation. Anything they do succeeds, and as soon as it is done they move on to the next thing, literally eager to move on.

John Updike, the American writer, has psoriasis. In his *Self-Consciousness: Memoirs* he devoted a whole 40 pages to describing his skin condition, saying that his creativity, the relentless desire to produce, was nothing but a parody of the painful overproduction in his skin.

Causes

The tendency to develop psoriasis is deeply rooted in the constitution and often inherited. It persists unchanged for life, even during phases when the skin is healthy. Under specific conditions the tendency to develop lesions in the skin increases and the disease then shows itself. This is referred to as raised 'endogenous eruption pressure'.

Factors that encourage psoriasis are:
- medicines such as beta-blockers, lithium, interferons
- alcohol
- purulent infections, e.g. tonsillitis
- weight gain and adiposity
- pregnancy
- stress, mental and nervous strain

The tissue changes due to psoriasis seen under the microscope show that the blood coming to the skin from metabolic processes in the centre has excessive power. People with psoriasis tend to have elevated uric acid, fat and sugar levels in the blood, a direct indication that metabolism is not adequately controlled. The factors which can aggravate psoriasis also suggest that with this condition one-sidedness is located in metabolism. It is interesting to note that the same signature can be found in the personality of someone with psoriasis. The will aspect is excessively powerful in the inner life and may go as far as a tremendous need to be active.

Treatment

Anthroposophical medical treatment of psoriasis is not easy, and this is also the case with any form of natural medicine. We tend to combine an approach to treatment designed to call up inner powers of self-healing with symptomatic treatment of the skin involving few side-effects. Symptoms are relieved in the short term, and the power which drives the psoriasis towards the skin from inside is reduced in the long term.

The liver is the central organ for metabolism. People with psoriasis not infrequently have sluggish liver function or even liver damage, or a disorder of the gall bladder and bile duct. If that is the case, liver and gall bladder need anthroposophical medical treatment with substances from the mineral and plant worlds (P). Quite frequently the intestine also shows imbalance in its resident microorganisms; certain yeasts may be present in excess. Treatment of this consists in strengthening the powers of digestion and improving the intestinal environment (P).

(See the section entitled 'Skin disease and yeasts in the intestine', pages 43–45.)

If patients overeat and are overweight or even obese, it will be necessary to reduce weight and change eating habits. The Schroth cure (in Germany) and F. X. Mayr treatment [in Austria, Tr.] are available for this. For the Schroth cure, a reduction diet is combined with whole-body packs. Dry white wine is usually permitted on days when fluids only are taken. People with psoriasis should take kvass (see section on diet earlier in this chapter) instead. For the F. X. Mayr cure, laxative treatment using bitter salts in the morning is followed by a 'gentle derivative diet' consisting of dry rolls and a cup of whole milk or yoghurt for breakfast and at midday. Intestinal function is stimulated by physical treatment of the abdomen, a method applied by physicians trained in Franz Xaver Mayr's method. The advantage of the Mayr cure is that patients will acquire new eating habits (e.g. chew each mouthful 40 times) for their normal diet, be able to enjoy their food more and so eat less and gain weight less quickly.

Chronic constipation (sluggish intestinal function) needs to be treated. Sauerkraut juice [health food stores or Internet, Tr.], ideally of Demeter quality, is excellent for this. Take half to one glass on an empty stomach in the morning (S). Like kvass, it provides the organism with lactic acid. This activates metabolism and cleanses. Mild psoriasis may certainly heal completely by just taking lactic acid products. An extract of red ant (Formica) taken internally has a similar effect, especially for lean people who tend to form deposits (P).

The use of fumaric acid cannot be considered part of natural medicine. High doses are needed to achieve an effect, and there may be side-effects. Fumaric acid treatment introduces something into the body in which it may (perhaps) be deficient; this is a principle used in conventional medicine (P).

As in the case of neurodermatitis, sunlight has an effect on psoriasis. The climate by the sea (sunlight and salt water) and in high mountain regions often helps to improve the condition. The Dead Sea should only be considered for very severe psoriasis. Powerful sunlight and a high percentage of salt in the water are a powerful measure, a 'climatic crowbar' which enforces healing at skin level but does not go deeper. The skin changes will often appear again in their old form just a few weeks after returning home.

For milder forms of psoriasis, external application of an ointment containing an extract from a barberry species (Rubisan ointment or cream, manuf. by DHU) is recommended (S). Other possibilities for external applications are Colchicum comp. Ointment[2], which contains autumn crocus (*Colchicum autumnale*) and greater celandine (*Chelidonium majus*) (P), and Birch Cream natural (less fat) or with beeswax (more fat) from Birken GmbH, with an extract of birch cork the active principle (S).

A medicinal plant for internal use is sarsaparilla (Sarsapsor, manuf. by Buerger) (P). In anthroposophical medicine, an extract of birch bark is injected under the skin, and a range of homoeopathic medicines may be used, their purpose being to give form to the metabolic sphere and limit the overweening anabolic powers in the psoriatic lesions (P).

One important medicine for psoriasis is potentized arsenic. It helps to direct the soul's activities towards the organ and metabolism (P). Autumn crocus is the vegetable arsenic. It is helpful if given in potentized form to people with psoriasis and elevated uric acid blood levels, thyroid and joint problems (P).

The natural spa water from Vetriolo, which is also used in the baths at Levico and Roncegno and contains much arsenic, has been successfully employed to treat psoriasis for over a hundred years. All three spas are near Trient in northern Italy (the anthroposophical clinic is in

Helpful	Unhelpful
sour milk products	spices: pepper, cloves, nutmeg, mustard, caraway, anise, cinnamon, paprika powder, also in all ready seasoned foods
lactic-fermented vegetables and vegetable juices	nuts: hazelnuts, walnuts, peanuts peel from citrus fruit, industrially processed lemon juice alcohol in any form
kvass	wine vinegar pork, pork sausages, much sugar, much coffee

Roncegno). Other important and polar opposite constituents of the water are iron and copper.

Evidently the most important thing is to advise someone with psoriasis to avoid any kind of food that 'heats up' metabolism. All 'sulphurous' foods must be avoided (e.g. mustard and pepper). Fats in the diet must be drastically reduced. Cod liver oil is a helpful food supplement, however, especially for old people with psoriasis and a tendency to develop arteriosclerosis. It is available in capsules. The table on the previous page shows helpful and unhelpful foods (based on the work of Dr Guenther Schaefer).

Contact dermatitis

This refers to eruptions caused by skin contact with a particular substance. A close look shows that two things contribute to the dermatitis – the substance coming in contact with the skin from outside, and the skin's readiness to react to it in a specific way. If the substance causes the organism to show an allergic reaction in the skin, we speak of 'allergic contact dermatitis'. If it has a toxic effect on the skin, causing irritation, the term used is 'toxic contact dermatitis'.

Substances in the environment that are liable to provoke an allergy in the human organism are known as 'allergens'. Nickel is one of the most common allergens today. Allergies to scents and preservatives are considered the most common causes of contact dermatitis due to body care products and cosmetics. Specific properties make a substance into an allergen. The compounds in arnica that cause allergies (sesquiterpene lactones) are very well known, for instance. They occur in the whole daisy family (Compositae), but the plants vary in how often they cause allergies. The capacity of a substance to provoke allergy is known as 'allergenicity'. Arnica is quite allergenic, for example, whereas chamomile and pot marigold have only minimal allergenicity.

It takes time for an allergy to develop. Daily contact with a substance may continue for years and then suddenly it is no longer tolerated. Chromate dermatitis of bricklayers and tilers characteristically develops after more than 10 or 20 years when there had been no problem before with the chromium salts in cement. Those affected find it hard to believe at first that they suddenly tolerate them no longer and develop dermatitis.

The organism needs at least a fortnight to develop an allergy. Following first contact with the allergen, inflammatory cells need this time to mature. The will lies dormant in them, as it were, to launch a massive attack on second contact. This period is called the 'sensitization phase'. It must pass before allergic contact dermatitis can develop. If dermatitis develops two weeks after first using a new body care product, the reason may be that the organism is sensitized without delay to one of the constituents.

Once sensitization has occurred and an allergy developed, any further contact with the substance concerned will result in allergic contact dermatitis. It does then, however, take at least half a day for the eruption to arise, sometimes it will even take three days. During this time, sensitized defence cells migrate from the blood vessels to the skin where they cause the inflammation.

Here's an example. Mrs X had a known nickel allergy and rightly avoided the metal for a long time. When her best friend got married she was firmly determined to wear her truly beautiful ear studs, even though they contained nickel. She put them on an hour before the wedding celebrations started, and enjoyed herself, wearing the beautiful studs. The next day the eruption started, weeping, with redness and swelling, yellowy crusts and severe itching, and she bore it patiently. When at least half a day passes between contact with the allergen and development of the eruption, we speak of a 'delayed-type' allergy. (Instant-type allergies also exist; they will be considered in connection with urticaria.)

It is advisable to avoid any substance to which one has become sensitive and which may cause allergic contact dermatitis. Nickel is an example of an avoidable allergen. German legislation permits only extremely low nickel content in objects for everyday use. It is different with arnica. It does have a certain allergenicity and should be avoided by individuals who are allergic to the plant. But it would be putting out the baby with the bath water if one were to ban arnica for external use in any ointment, cream, lotion or gel. The plant is most valuable and effective, and this fully makes up for the allergenicity.

If contact dermatitis has developed and the allergen comes in contact with the skin again and again, the eruption may become highly acute and spread also to regions of the body where contact with the allergen did not occur.

An example. Open ulcers may develop on the lower legs with varicose veins, and may persist for months. They are treated daily with a wound-healing ointment; this will not infrequently cause an allergy to a constituent of the ointment, and contact dermatitis develops. If the cause is not identified and the same ointment continues to be used, the dermatitic lesions may spread from the lower legs to the face, backs of hands and forearms, or to the whole of the back.

If a causal connection between dermatitis and a specific substance is suspected, one can apply a specific concentration of it in vaseline or water to the skin and cover it with a plaster. This is the patch or epicutaneous test. The plaster stays in place for 24 hours before it is removed and the skin area assessed for the first time. It is looked at a second time after 48 and if necessary also a third time after 72 hours. In principle, any substance can be skin tested like this. It is customary to test the 24 most common allergens en bloc.

It is, however, important not to do the test until the dermatitis has gone. If it has not, and the whole skin organ is still on alert, it can happen that the skin reacts with irritation to substances to which it is not actually allergic. The test results may thus be unreliable if the epicutaneous test is done too soon after an acute contact dermatitis. In any case, the results must be compared with the observations which physician and patient made on the dermatitis; this means they have to be interpreted. This makes the distinction between genuine allergies, where test result and the history preceding the dermatitis agree, and 'falsely positive' reactions (usually due to skin irritation). The latter are of no importance where the dermatitis in question is concerned.

People who have reacted to scents in the epicutaneous test so that one must assume them to have an allergy to scent, are generally advised by dermatologists to avoid all scented body care products, cosmetics and medicines. In practice it has been found with the use of natural cosmetics scented with natural essential oils that people with scent allergies tolerate these well. This has recently been confirmed in a trial where a relatively large number of people allergic to scents were tested systematically. The solution to the contradiction is that scents in the usual body care products are pure compounds isolated from natural essential oils, or synthetic compounds. These are not always

81

well tolerated. The natural essential oils used in natural cosmetics (e.g. those produced by Weleda and Wala) are complex compositions and these are generally well tolerated.

This is a good example to show that substances in our environment which do not come from the shared evolution of nature and man always impose a strain on the human organism.

Allergic contact dermatitis can determine someone's destiny at the occupational level. Having become sensitized to chromium salts, the above-mentioned tiler will have to avoid all further contact with cement, and that means he can no longer stay in the same job. Once a connection has been established between a skin eruption and contact with materials used in one's occupation, all measures taken to achieve a cure, including retraining in another occupation where the work place is clean and dry, are paid for by the employer's organization in Germany. There are many measures that can be taken to prevent skin diseases (see under 'Hand dermatitis' on p. 85). Yet in spite of this, contact allergies are the commonest causes of occupational disease.

The tendency to develop an allergy to something and get dermatitis following skin contact varies greatly between people. It often runs in families, which means it is hereditary. Nickel allergy often occurs in conjunction with neurodermatitis, hay fever and asthma, for example. Liability to develop dermatitis also varies in one and the same person at different stages of life. It is quite often greater in times of mental and nervous strain. Problems at work, marital strife, a tiff with one's best friend can go hand in hand with a shaving lotion or eye cream proving intolerable. On the other hand there is a constitutional, inherited type of skin which does not stand up to much stress. This is skin which tends to be dry, with frequent hand washing, especially in winter, causing dryness and letting allergens penetrate more quickly to deeper skin layers.

Apart from allergic contact dermatitis, another form arises through contact with skin irritants that damage the epidermis, which may lead to toxic contact dermatitis. Allergic and toxic contact dermatitis look the same. It needs the art of the dermatologist to establish the cause in each case. A typical dermatitis due to toxic factors may develop, for instance, when a car mechanic uses organic solvents (benzene or alcohol, for instance) to clean his oily hands. The solvents destroy the protective layer of fat on the skin and irritate the skin or even inflame it. In everyday life, irritant and drying actions coming from outside may be quite mild, but frequent exposure does ultimately lead to dermatitis.

Housewives' dermatitis is an example. It develops due to water, washing up liquids and cleaning agents used in the home, doing laundry, etc.

Toxic and allergic elements may come together in causing contact dermatitis. If a painter tends to have a dry skin, cleaning paint off his hands using an aggressive paste can cause the backs of the hands to grow dry and irritated. Once the skin has been damaged in this way, an allergen, for instance a substance in one of the paints, can penetrate more quickly to deeper layers in the epidermis and trigger sensitization. This is called a 'two-stage dermatitis'. The toxic contact dermatitis of the first stage becomes allergic contact dermatitis as sensitization to a substance develops in the second stage.

As a rule, sunlight soothes dermatitis. It may happen, however, that a substance on the skin only develops its allergizing or irritant effect on exposure to sunlight. If you lie in a freshly mown meadow exposing your skin to the sun, it can happen that plant saps, especially from a member of the carrot family (Umbelliferae) such as hogweed, combines with the sunlight to create a skin eruption. This is known as 'meadow grass dermatitis'. Following contact with the sap from leaves and stems it tends to develop in stripes and may also produce vesicles. Some of the substances used in perfumes can also cause phototoxic contact dermatitis in sunlight if applied directly to the skin. Photo-allergic contact dermatitis is much rarer. They can be triggered by light-protective factors in sun creams, etc. Medicines reaching the skin from inside via the blood, such as some diuretics, can also cause this dermatitis.

As the name implies, the substance reaching the skin from outside is usually of prime importance with contact dermatitis. This also justifies the use of cortisol (see section on cortisol on p. 53). It has powerful symptomatic actions and will quickly relieve symptoms such as pruritus. If the trigger is known to come from outside, this must be avoided, and a suitable cortisol product may be used with confidence (P). If it is not quite so important to the patient to get rid of the dermatitis quickly, the following measures are recommended for acute contact dermatitis:

- during the weeping stage – moist compresses with an infusion of Indian tea or oak bark (tannins), mallow and chamomile (anti-inflammatory) (S).
- during the dry, reddened stage – Calendula Baby Cream[1] or soft zinc paste, during the day olive oil, Almond Intensive Facial Cream[1] or Halicar Ointment [DHU, Germany, Tr.]; Rosatum Ointment[2] (fatty) or Wund- und Brandgel[2] (gel for treating wounds and burns) are also suitable (S).
- during the dry stage, with the redness getting less – only ointments that provide fat, as listed above) during the day (S).

It is also helpful to take Calcium carbonicum/Cortex quercus Pilules[2] in addition, 10 pilules before meals 2–5 times/day (S). If the tendency to develop dermatitis is marked, your physician will try and reduce this by treating you constitutionally with anthroposophical medicines (P).

Dermatitis on the eyelids (palpebral dermatitis)

An eruption in the region of the eyes, with redness, more or less marked swelling and fine scales is particularly unpleasant as it is very visible and also tends to be very itchy. In most cases it reflects a constitutional tendency to develop neurodermatitis and nervous tension. People consider the eyes to be their most important sense organ; you guard things of special value to you 'like the apple of your eye'.

The first severe dermatitis of the eyelids the author saw at a dermatological clinic was in a student who studied during the day, going to lectures, and earned the money he needed for this by working as a taxi driver by night. The excessive strain on the eyes, and indeed the whole nervous system, was perfectly evident in this case.

Eczema of the eyelids may, however, also point to intolerance of a facial or hair care product. When hair care products are used that irritate the skin, it is often the case that a reaction develops not in the more robust skin of the scalp but in neighbouring areas – throat, back of neck, forehead, and of course also the area around the eyes. All skin and hair care products must be tested for tolerance. Hair care products often cannot be said to be skin-tolerated because they tend to be aggressive. Gentle alternatives are the Weleda and Wala products, as they cause very little irritation.

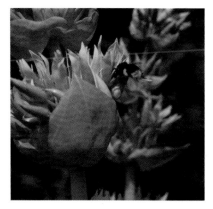

Yellow gentian

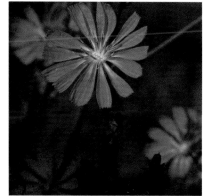

Chicory

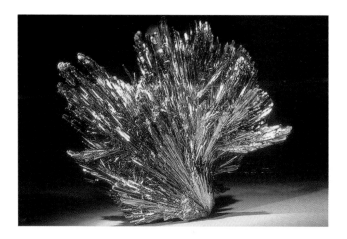

Antimonite

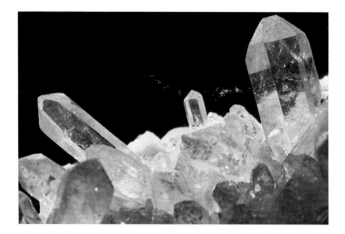

Rock crystal

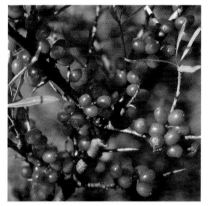

Sea buckthorn

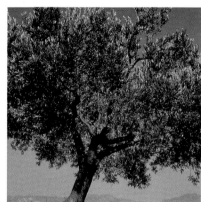

Olive tree

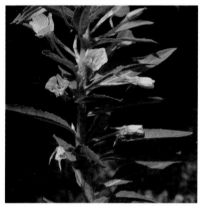

Evening primrose

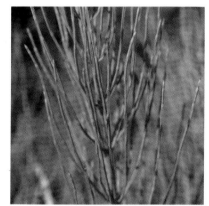

Horsetail

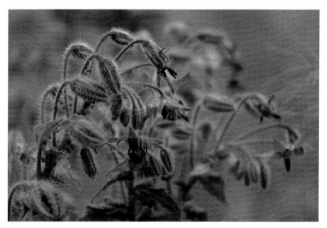

Borage

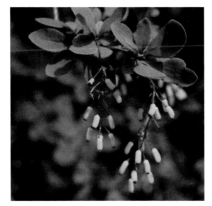

Barberry

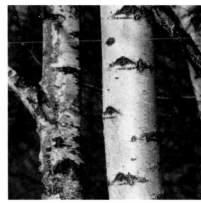

Birch bark

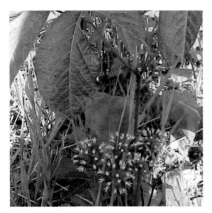

Sarsaparilla

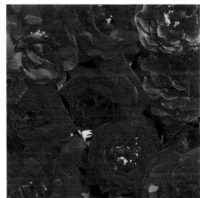

Roses

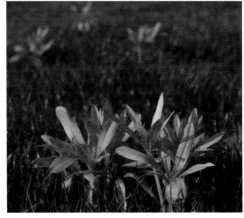

Autumn crocus

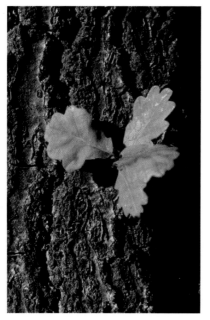

Oak

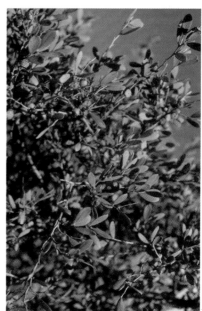

Tea tree

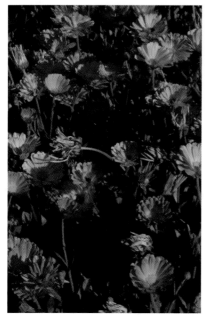

Pot marigold

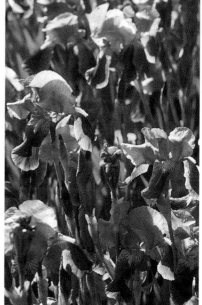

Iris

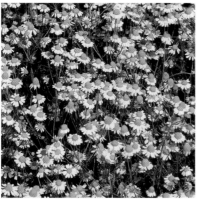

Chamomile

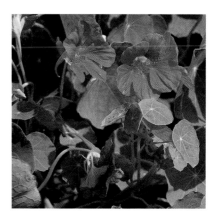

Nasturtium

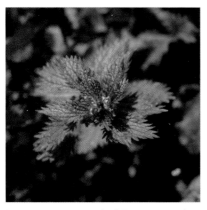

Lesser stinging nettle (Urtica urens)

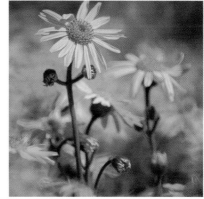

Arnica

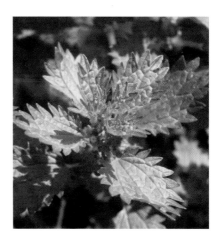

Greater stinging nettle (Urtica dioica)

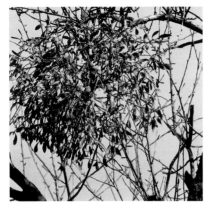

Mistletoe

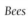

Bees

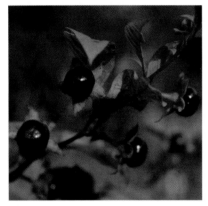

Deadly nightshade

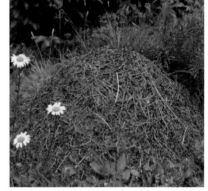

Ant heap

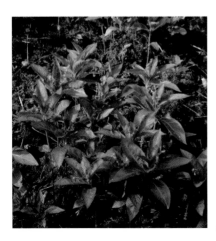

Dog's mercury

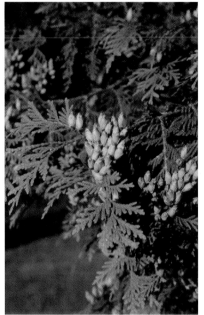

Arbor vitae

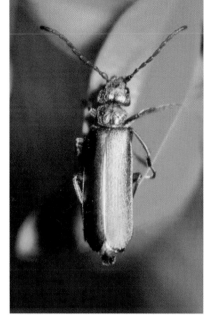

'Spanish fly'

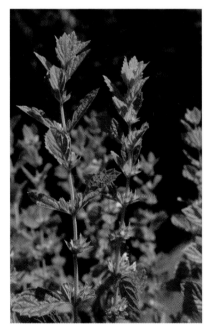

Lemon balm

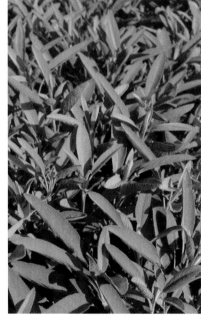

Sage

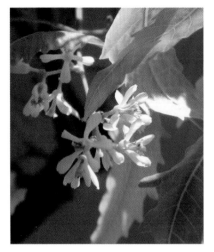

Flowering neem tree

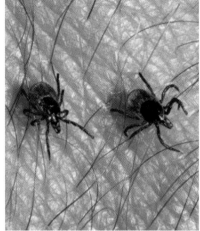

Ticks

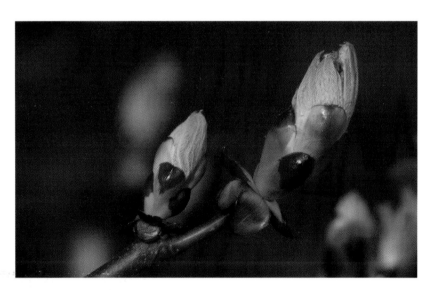

Horse chestnut buds

In rare cases, eczema of the eyelids may reflect a functional weakness in the liver; this calls for treatment of the liver using medicinal herbs (P).

If the area around the eyes is much swollen and also red and inflamed, moist compresses with Indian tea are helpful (S). Dr Hauschka's Augenfrische pads are also helpful (S). Or you may use Calendula Baby Cream[1] (contains zinc) at night and Antimonite 0.4% Ointment[1] during the day (S). If the skin is mainly dry and scaly, use Antimonite 0.4% Ointment on its own several times a day (S). Rosatum Heilsalbe[2] (wound healing ointment) is also suitable in this case (S).

Hand dermatitis

Eruptions on the hands are quite common but vary greatly in appearance and causes. Let us first consider the differences in appearance. The dermatitis is often limited to the palms and sides of fingers. Itching, sometimes painful small vesicles come up at intervals; they may join up in more extensive areas that weep and form crusts, then dry up, with flaky skin, before they disappear. The soles and sides of the feet may also be affected, though this is much more uncommon. The condition is also referred to as 'dyshidrotic dermatitis' which means that the management of fluids in the skin is not functioning properly.

Another form is hyperkeratotic dermatitis. Again the palms are affected, but this time with a tendency of the epidermis to harden. Cornified plaques develop over larger areas or in isolation, sometimes reddened due to inflammation. The cracks which develop in the plaques due to movement (rhagades) are very painful and may get infected.

The causes of hand dermatitis are most often internal, due to the individual constitution. It is especially in identifying the causes of hand dermatitis that the physician's knowledge of essential human nature plays a major role. To put it bluntly, in natural medicine, and especially also anthroposophical medicine, the importance of the individual disposition, the tendency towards dermatitis, ranks high. In conventional dermatology, external causes are generally given particular consideration. Both approaches are reasonable, and the physician must use both of them in looking for the causes in a given case.

Internal causes of hand dermatitis may be
- atopic skin diathesis
- psoriasis
- functional weakness of internal organs (liver, kidneys, intestine).

External causes may be
- fungal infection
- allergic contact dermatitis
- toxic contact dermatitis.

A physician often sees a particular type of personality among people with dyshidrotic dermatitis whose palms dissolve for a time, with weeping, inflamed vesicles appearing on the palms. They include female hairdressers and nurses, who show sensitivity and patiently listen to the cares of their customers and worries of patients. The things they are told affect them; they will often not be able to forget them that quickly. This shows them to be thin-skinned. The dissolving skin of the palms, the main area of contact with the world in everything we do, gives a picture at the organic level of the problem of keeping the world out. These women are too open to the world around them.

Weeping hand dermatitis at the acute vesicular stage dries up quickly if you apply Foot Balm[1] overnight, wearing cotton gloves (S). Hand baths in a decoction of oak bark or Tannolact (manuf. by Galderma), a synthetic tannin, soothe the weeping inflammation (S). Dry hand dermatitis and especially the type that tends to grow cornified improve with Antimonite 0.4% ointment[1], applied at least twice a day (S). Keloid Gel[2] is effective where hardening is severe (S). If the hands need care that provides them with fat, Dr Hauschka Hand Cream or Sea Buckthorn Hand Cream[1] are recommended (S). Painful cracks heal quickly with applications of Wecesin Powder[1] covered over with a plaster (S).

If external causes can be largely excluded and the dermatitis gets worse after eating sweets, for instance, or taking alcohol, it will be necessary to treat a possible weakness in the digestive system (P). Dyshidrotic dermatitis with episodes when weeping vesicles appear may indicate that the fluid organism of the individual concerned is not functioning properly. This calls for horsetail, using a herbal product (or tea) or a potentized form of it (P). Someone with this type of dermatitis who is also too 'thin-skinned' mentally can be helped to grow a 'thicker skin' using potentized medicines (P). Calcium carbonicum/ Cortex quercus Pilules[2], 10 pilules 2–5 times daily before meals, will always soothe the inflammation (S).

People whose hand dermatitis is partly or wholly due to substances used at work or in the household should take note of the following:

- Avoid skin contact with all harmful substances.
- Wash hands in lukewarm water, using unscented soap; avoid brushes and aggressive cleaners; rinse soap off well; dry thoroughly, then apply skin-care cream.
- Take off rings when doing housework, as cleaning agents can collect under them and damage the skin.
- Use washing machine and dishwasher.
- Wear protective PVC gloves. Rubber increases the risk of sensitization.
- Wear cotton gloves under the PVC ones; this absorbs the sweat.
- Wear protective gloves when preparing citrus fruit, tomatoes or potatoes in the kitchen.
- Every time the skin goes dry, apply hand creams during the day and rich ointments at night (under cotton gloves obtainable from chemists or drugstores).

Stasis dermatitis

Stasis dermatitis most commonly affects the lower leg, above the ankle. Highly acute forms are weeping, chronic forms are dry and scaling and may cause severe pruritus. Especially in the evenings, when people with healthy skins enjoy resting from their work, the pruritus can prove unbearable and often will not stop for the individual concerned for the first half of the night after going to bed.

This dermatitis gives a rough hint of the cause by its localization. Metabolism is often sluggish, with a need to eliminate metabolic waste via the skin. Varicose veins are a special case here. Blood in stasis in the varicose veins causes water to collect in the tissues (oedema); towards evening the lower part of the leg swells up. This changes the metabolic situation in the skin, and the dermatitis develops. If varicose veins have resulted in ulcers in the lower legs, moist discharges from these and the ointments used day after day for long periods finally cause the dermatitis. Sensitization to a constituent of one of the ointments used often plays a role in the development of the condition (see under Contact dermatitis, pages 79–84). The dermatitis tends to develop in the immediate vicinity of the ulceration.

Treatment should serve to relieve and stimulate metabolism. The diet should include little sugar and protein (i.e. meat, dairy produce, eggs); overweight must be reduced. Intestines, liver and/or kidneys may need medical treatment (P). The treatment for varicose veins is considered in a separate section (pages 151–155).

If inflammation is severe, use external combination treatment. During the night, a preparation containing zinc oxide will soothe; Calendula Baby Cream[1] or soft zinc paste may be used for this. It is possible to get zinc paste without lanolin at a pharmacy. Zinc oxide has a drying action and this must be made up for by using an ointment containing fat during the day. Quercus Ointment[2] is suitable for this (S). Calcium carbonicum/Cortex quercus Pilules[2] taken by mouth will calm the inflammatory reaction, 10 pilules 2–5 times a day before meals (S).

Dermatitis in the genital and anal region

Irritation (pruritus) tends to dominate the picture, often with no visible skin changes. Irritation in the genital region and in the gluteal fold around the anus is such a problem to people that they cannot enjoy the rest and peacefulness normal for the evening, when the soul needs to breathe out. Night-time sleep may also prove difficult; the soul is caught up, as it were, in those skin areas and cannot come free. The problem tends to appear more in the genital region for women and the anal region for men. If inflammatory changes develop in the skin, they appear as redness, thickening and dry scaliness in the external genitalia of women (the vulva). Fissures often develop around the anus in both genders. Anal dermatitis can become weeping in the gluteal fold if inflammation is severe. Genital dermatitis is rare in males.

This type of dermatitis is generally a special variant of neuro-dermatitis and worse under stress. Thus a woman with three young children, tall and slim, finds everyday life a struggle; her husband travels for his firm and is only at home at weekends. The constant stress during the day results in her being too much awake in the neurosensory sphere, and in a 'short circuit' effect powers of conscious awareness mediated by the nerves 'strike' at the centre of metabolism. This is the sphere of reproduction, the highest function in the metabolic system. The skin in the genital region, normally asleep to some degree, comes awake and over-awake and pruritus develops. Inflammatory changes develop in the skin with dermatitis through the blood's attempt at self-healing; it seeks to counterbalance overweening processes in the nerves and overshoots the mark in the process.

Another common cause is sluggish liver function causing dermatitis in the anal rather than the genital region. A sluggish liver with reduced vitality slows down the blood's inherent mobility; the blood then stays longer in the venous system of the minor pelvis than is healthy. This changes the metabolic situation of the skin in the gluteal fold, which is then latently 'over-juiced'; piles may also develop (see section on Haemorrhoids, pages 155–157). Anal dermatitis and piles thus often appear together.

Baths can be helpful in treating genital and anal dermatitis. A bath with Lavender Relaxing Bath Milk[1] provides general warmth and relaxation, especially for genital dermatitis with neurodermatitis in the background (S). Sulphur baths may be tried to get the often highly chronic dermatitis moving (P). If the lesions are weeping, the tannin in an oak bark decoction or Tannolact (manuf. by Galderma) may be helpful (S). Calendula Baby Cream[1] is often wonderfully soothing if there is inflammation and a tendency for lesions to weep (S); the effect is largely due to the zinc content of the product. If eczematous lesions threaten to become weeping, a strip of gauze (an opened-up non-sterile gauze pad, 10 × 10 cm) may be placed in the gluteal fold after applying the cream. It acts like a wick in soaking up the moisture. Foot Balm[1] is effective because of its alumina content combined with an extract of myrrh (S). Hamamelis comp. Ointment[1], Stibium metallicum prep. 0.4% Ointment[1] and Quercus Ointment[2/1] contain fats and are particularly suitable for treating anal dermatitis (S). Neurodermatitis of the vulva is relieved with Argentum metallicum prep. 0.4% Ointment[1] or Bismutum/Stibium Ointment[1] (S).

For genital dermatitis with neurodermatitis in the background it is necessary to strengthen vitality by taking potentized silver (Argentum) internally (P). Reducing the nervous strain (e.g. by taking a holiday) will often improve the situation. Anal dermatitis with weak liver function improves if Fragaria/Vitis comp. Tablets[1] and Achillea comp. dil. drops[1] are taken by mouth (P).

Intertrigo

Intertrigo develops due to skin irritation in areas where skin meets skin – underarm, in the inguinal and genital regions, in the gluteal fold, and in corpulent people also in the abdominal fold and in women under the breasts. A redness develops which sharply defines the areas of skin-to-skin contact. The upper epidermis may become macerated (softened) and separate from the rest. This is usually accompanied by pruritus and burning pain, and the area may weep and develop an unpleasant smell.

The causes of intertrigo are friction between skin and skin or through clothing. Other external causes are sweat which cannot evaporate and macerates the skin, and overweight. The inflamed, embattled, over-juiced skin is susceptible to excessive bacterial growth and also yeast infection (candida). In cases of obesity it is perfectly obvious that the metabolism is overburdened, but less evident metabolic disorders, including diabetes, can contribute to intertrigo developing from the inside.

Milder degrees of skin irritation will improve quickly with Calendula Baby Cream[1], which contains zinc oxide (S). Severe inflammation with bacterial and yeast infection may respond to Birch Cream Natural (manuf. by Birken GmbH) (S). It contains betulin which acts against bacteria and yeasts. Baths with an oak bark decoction or Tannolact powder (manuf. by Galderma), both containing tannins, encourage healing (S). If the condition is persistent and severe, use gentian violet 0.5% in aqueous solution (obtainable from pharmacies) (S). It is best to use disposable gloves when applying it as it stains the skin, patting it on with a pad of cotton wool and then using a hairdryer to dry it. Do this once a day for three days and then change to Calendula Baby Cream[1]. Dulcamara/Lysimachia Drops[1] may be taken by mouth, 10–20 drops three times daily before meals (S).

Nappy/diaper rash

The gluteal fold and front part of the nappy region are generally much reddened; sometimes the skin in the whole nappy region is inflamed. The signs of yeast infection are small red nodules and plaques scattered over the healthy surrounding skin. Final confirmation only comes if the physician takes scrapings for a laboratory culture.

Baby skin is put under great stress in the nappy or diaper region. The moisture from urine and stools makes the skin swell and dry out; if digestive disorders make the stools 'acrid', this means an additional attack on the skin. Yeasts also like to grow in the moist warmth of a well-wrapped baby bottom, where air tends to be excluded. Infants with dry skin and a tendency to develop neurodermatitis are most easily affected. The tendency to have dermatitis increases in all infants when they are teething. The tooth erupts through the oral mucosa from inside to the outside and this goes in the same direction as a skin eruption. This is why nappy or diaper rash is also more common in teething infants.

If disposables have been used so far, change to fabric nappies or diapers and vice versa. The change may bring improvement by itself. Fabric nappies are a bit more airy, whereas disposables are more absorbent. To limit skin dryness, bathe the baby only once a week. The diaper region should never be washed with water. Simply cleanse the skin with Calendula Baby Oil[1] or pure olive oil on cotton wool or disposable wipes. It is wonderful and a great benefit for the skin in the nappy region if the child can be left without clothes on in a warm room or out of doors in warm weather. Protect and care for the skin with Calendula Baby Cream[1]. Yeast infections are removed with a pigment such as gentian violet 0.5% in aqueous solution. Apply the brilliant violet solution on cotton wool once a day for three successive days and then change to Calendula Baby Cream[1] (S). Another external application that may be used to treat nappy/diaper rash with or without yeast infection is Birch Cream (manuf. by Birken GmbH). If the yeast comes from the child's intestine (stool test), the intestine needs to be treated with herbal and potentized medicines (P).

Hypericum Oil is excellent in caring for the skin in the nappy region and for nappy rash. St John's wort (*Hypericum perforatum*) contains hypericin (antidepressant action) and hyperforin (antibacterial and anti-inflammatory actions); the last of these is important for external use. It develops in the flowering and fruiting region of the plant under the influence of summer light and heat. To make hypericum oil, you have to exclude light. Fill either a stoneware container with close-fitting lid or a brown glass bottle one quarter full with minced-up flowers and/or ground-up fruit capsules, add olive oil to the top and leave to stand for four weeks, shaking occasionally. Strain through a fine sieve or a cloth and store in brown glass bottles with tight-fitting tops. Recommended ready-made oils are Hypericum 25% Oil[2] (from the flowers) and Hypericum herba 5% Oil[2] (from the leaves). It may be used undiluted to cleanse the nappy region. For nappy/diaper rash, use 10% of it in soft zinc paste (Pasta zinci mollis) (S).

Dermatitis in the elderly

Dry skin creates fine cracks similar to the hairline cracks in bone china. These can get inflamed and cause dry dermatitis. Localization is mainly in the extremities. If there is more of an inner disposition for dermatitis, the whole skin may be covered with small red, scaling plaques or itching nodules. Pruritus is often the worst part of dermatitis in the elderly, not uncommonly worse than the suffering due to more severe pain. The skin of older people may also itch without anything showing on the outside. Pruritus in old age points to excessive powers of conscious awareness in the skin; these come free as part of the ageing process at the organic level.

The function of the sebaceous glands is greatly reduced in all older people; little sebum then reaches the skin, which makes it more dry. The lowest density of sebum is found in the skin on the arms and legs; this is why the skin is most likely to go dry there. Older people often tend to wash more often and more intensively, not adapting their washing habits to the dryness of their skin. Swimming in indoor pools and saunas in winter make particular demands on the skin of older people.

However, not only does the skin show regression of anabolic function in old age; the internal organs (liver and kidneys) also show reduced metabolic activity. Their functions of detoxication and elimination are no longer adequate, and the skin must take on more than enough of them. As a result it 'flowers' into dermatitis. Old age also means a growing tendency to become sclerotic, and this affects the whole organism. Loss of vitality at the organic level contrasts with increased activity at the level of soul and spirit. The wisdom of old people can serve as evidence of this.

As a first step, skin care must provide the needed fat. It is advisable to use replenishing skin care at night, before going to bed, so that one's outer garments do not get greasy. Depending on the amount of fat needed, use Skin Food[1], Cold Cream[1] or Rosatum Heilsalbe[2] (ointment) (S). If there is more marked skin irritation, washing down with water and vinegar and then applying chamomile flower oil (Chamomile flower 10%, Oil[2]) or Dr Hauschka Lavender Body Oil may be helpful (S). Severe dermatitis of old age will also need internal treatment. Apart from an extract of birch bark (P), birch leaf tea or Birch Elixir[1] (S) will balance out sluggish metabolism internally and the tendency to sclerosis in the skin. Red ant in homoeopathic potencies taken by mouth will also activate the metabolism (P). Herbal medicines may also be needed to stimulate liver and kidney functions (P). Nierentonikum[2] (kidney tonic) is recommended for this (S).

Lichen planus

Lichen planus, sometimes also called lichen ruber planus, has its name from tiny, itching nodules (papules) spreading individually or merging with others which makes them look like lichen. Preferred sites are the insides of wrists and forearms, the sides of ankle joints, the skin above the sacrum (lower back) and the genital area. The lichen may also appear on the oral mucosa (inner lining of the mouth), typically as netlike, whitish linear lesions on the insides of the cheeks. Pruritus is the main symptom and usually intense; it may also affect healthy skin areas. Lichen planus first develops mainly at ages 20 to 60 and tends to be chronic.

The causes are often nerve strain. Chemically produced medicines may also trigger the condition. A family man aged 35 was a very successful head of department in an electronics firm. He and his wife had planned and built a house; when the expensive, made-to-measure built-in kitchen units were delivered, they turned out to be 50 cm larger than ordered. Completion and the move to the new house were delayed for weeks, a problem as they had already given notice for the flat which they had rented until then. At this point, the tall, slender, wide-awake man developed severely itching papules on the wrists.

The cause in the sphere of nerves and senses is made visible in the papules which are quite hard and very itchy. The nervous tension of everyday life − 'it nerves me' − turns into hardening in the skin and excessive wakefulness − the pruritus.

Treatment with the means available in anthroposophical medicine needs patience. It sometimes takes months to achieve real success, but relief and healing are certainly possible. An anthroposophical physician will, for example, use a combination of antimony and arsenic in potentized form to try and take the excessive soul activity at the level of nerves and senses down into metabolism (P). Stibium metallicum prep. 0.4% Ointment[1] is often helpful (S).

Seborrhoeic dermatitis

Seborrhoea means 'flow of sebum'. Seborrhoeic dermatitis is therefore an eruption found mainly in skin areas with high density of sebaceous glands, so that the skin surface is greasier − scalp, eyebrows, middle parts of forehead, nose and adjacent parts of the face, and in the 'sweat channels' on the front and back of the trunk.

The spots, usually not very red, have a brown tinge to them. The skin does not thicken. Inflammation of the scalp can lead to loss of hair, but it will grow again once the dermatitis has gone.

A yeast (*Pityrosporum ovale*) is often present in greater density than on healthy skin. It is suspected that it plays a role in the development of the condition. But an inherited tendency to greasy skin also has a part in it. Just as there is inherited dry skin tending towards neuro-dermatitis, so greasy skin means a tendency to develop seborrhoeic dermatitis, acne and rosacea.

People with seborrhoeic dermatitis quite often show a slowing down in liver function. At the same time the amount of yeasts in the intestine may be increased. There is no outward connection between yeasts on the skin and yeasts in the intestines; they are quite different species. But there is an inner connection in so far as the organism's powers to impose form are inadequate in both terrains – skin and intestine. Foreign life can then take up the space with a density and intensity that goes beyond the norm.

Helpful external measures reduce the excess yeast – purified coal tar, wood tars, shale oil, and also sulphur (as a shampoo on the head, zinc suspension [cala-mine lotion, Tr.] or zinc paste in other akin areas) (P). Tea tree oil also combats fungi such as yeast, but can be irritant and must be stopped immediately if the skin reddens progressively (S).

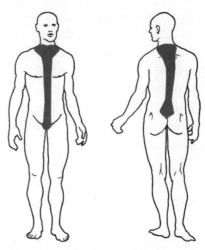

Sweat channels, front and back

Weekly baths, with horsetail decoction or sulphur added, depending on one's constitution, can activate metabolism internally and thus relieve the skin (P). If your physician finds indications of a minor weakness in liver function, this calls for herbal medical treatment for the liver (P).

Acne

Together with neurodermatitis and psoriasis, acne is one of the most common skin conditions. The situation of the human organism in puberty is typical for ordinary acne. Starting at 10 to 14 and completed at 18 or 19 years of age, the growing individual develops sexual maturity. Hormone levels need to settle, with the ratio of male to female hormones also highly individual within one of the genders. This is just a specific aspect of the metabolic process. The whole metabolism matures during those years.

The same holds true for the psyche. The opposite sex is taken note of, ideals grasped, individuality develops. Going through a stage of mood changes, growing inwardness, powerful feelings, negativity and uncertainty in the social sphere, the young person arrives at an individual way of dealing with the environment, his or her own way of responsibly shaping life and developing friendships. In between one will tend to see mild chaos in the psyche, which is part of the process of gaining adulthood. This is reflected in the body, where the changes in metabolism may temporarily enter into a state of 'ferment'. This 'fermenting metabolism' seeks to find its own way to the outside; we get a picture of this in the inflamed acne pustule. Metabolic processes that are still at an awkward stage must be taken hold of in a new way and given form.

Unfortunately it almost always happens in the face, less frequently also around the neckline and on the upper back. This aggravates the young person's insecurity. He lives in inner shifts and changes, lacking balance; looking in the mirror he sees his spotty face like a confirmation of his inner situation. This makes acne in puberty a skin condition which will no doubt disappear one day but right now is a real problem – a pain.

The situation in puberty also tells us in which direction to look for the causes of adult acne. If a woman of about 30 is still suffering from acne, a physician working with natural medicine will find it worth while to look for 'residual puberty' in the metabolic sphere, a corner in the organism that was not wholly taken hold of and reshaped in puberty.

Stress can aggravate acne. The number of pustules tends to increase shortly before or during the menstrual period. Acne generally gets worse in winter, as metabolism is more sluggish in that season, whereas the summer sun improves the situation. Powerful sun can, however, also have a bad effect. Roughly speaking we can say that acne is more likely to develop in skin with a hereditary tendency to seborrhoea (sebum flow). But people with dry skin can also develop acne. Certain medicinal products (e.g. vitamin B, iodine) may trigger acne if taken. From the outside, care products based on mineral oils (vaseline, paraffin) may have a negative influence.

The secretion of sebum from sebaceous glands is stimulated by male hormone. In puberty the glands produce more sebum. On the other hand the fact that the glands share their exit pores with those of fine hairs means that there is increased cornification. Horn and sebum combine in a plug (comedo). If this is black (blackhead), the colour is due to melanocytic pigment. Specific microorganisms in the skin may multiply in the blocked-up sebum, with fatty acids released from their metabolism. Those fatty acids irritate the surrounding tissues in the dermis and cause inflammation. Spots (papules) develop, then pustules with their yellow heads of pus.

If the skin is very greasy and the pustules are 'juicy', painting on Calendula Essence, 20%[1] in zinc suspension [calamine lotion] overnight (S) is soothing. Pot marigold (*Calendula officinalis*) is the medicinal plant for all purulent processes in the skin. Spots should only be squeezed cautiously, with clean fingers, once a yellow head has formed, which means that they are 'ripe'. Suitable products for skin care with acne are Iris Cleansing Lotion[1] (on cotton wool for cleansing in the mornings and at night) and Iris Facial Toner[1] (to dab on to the spots in between times) (S). A facial steam bath with chamomile tea once or twice a week will soften the blackheads and reduce inflammation in spots and pustules (S). Follow with an Almond Oil[1] face pack or Almond Facial Masque[1], which work in the same direction (S). If inflammation is more severe and the skin more greasy, it is helpful to apply a pack with Luvos Heilerde 1 or 2 (natural loess, manuf. by Luvos) after the steam bath. Mix the loess with water to a paste and apply to the whole face; leave to act for up to 30 minutes (S).

Wala offer a lotion, steam bath and face mask for the treatment of acne (S). One characteristic medicinal agent in these is nasturtium (*Tropaeolum majus*), a plant of sulphurous nature which is able to vitalize skin metabolism. Cleanse the face with Dr Hauschka Cleansing Cream before using the lotion. If the skin on the face is inclined to be greasy, a face oil may certainly be used during the day. It soothes the hyperactive sebaceous glands, so one is 'pouring oil on to troubled waters', as it were.

As a dermatologist, I would certainly recommend that a cosmetician is also consulted. She can teach acne patients specific methods and discuss practical aspects with them. Loving care will also help to restore the self-esteem which has often suffered from those extensive inflamed areas in the face. Of course, it should be a cosmetician who truly works with love and has a light hand, not merely wanting to clear out every spotty bit of the face thoroughly and completely.

Internal treatment of acne using anthroposophical medicines serves to harmonize metabolism and activate it in areas where it has grown sluggish. Sulphur and phosphorus, given by mouth in homoeopathic preparations, are helpful in giving impulses to and tightening up metabolism (P). Quartz in homoeopathic potency takes care of the balance between metabolism and skin; it calms inflammation the way sand puts out a fire (P). Homoeopathic iron preparations help to mature metabolism and assist the growing-up process altogether; this metal makes the young person 'ready for earth' (P).

Acne in someone with weak liver function will often improve with herbal medical treatment of the liver (P). Other organic spheres must also be taken into account. Any tendency to constipation must be corrected to establish regular daily stools (S). Acne Capsules[2] regulate metabolism quite generally (S). If the feet tend to be cold, this indicates that the whole metabolism needs to be warmed through. A copper ointment (Cuprum metallicum prep. 0.4% Ointment[1] or Red Copper Ointment[2]) applied thinly to the feet and lower legs at night is helpful in this case (S).

Irregular menses and menstrual pain also need to be treated (P). It may be said in very general terms that once the cycle is fully established, normal menstruation with no spasms of pain is a process of elimination in the pelvis which means there is no need to eliminate via acne pustules at the other end of the organism, in the face.

Acne of puberty in young women is often treated with the antibaby (contraceptive) pill which contains much oestrogen. This shifts the balance between female and male hormones in favour of the former. The male hormones which aggravate the acne lose importance. The 'pill' is often effective in treating acne in this way, but there are drawbacks as well. It can happen that the acne comes up again when the 'pill' is stopped in the late twenties, say because the woman and her partner want to have a child. A hormonal rhythm imposed from outside at an early stage prevented the natural development of functions in this sphere of the female organism, and there is now need to catch up. A bit of puberty has persisted into adulthood at the organic level. On the other hand taking synthetic hormones for years, or even decades, can put a strain on the liver. The liver has to break these substances down and this can in the long run reduce its metabolic powers. This will in turn make the acne worse; acne in puberty then leads to adult acne years later.

Some patients find that certain foods aggravate their acne; for others there is no connection between acne and diet. Acne sufferers should test for themselves if they get more spots from eating particular foods.

The foods in question are chocolate, sweets, refined sugar, white flour, pork, crisps, fatty foods (e.g. mayonnaise), hard cheeses with a high fat content, nuts, citrus fruit. The effect that the diet has on the skin condition depends on whether or not individuals have sluggish liver function, often combined with weak digestion.

Rosacea

Acne and rosacea have some things in common. They are more likely to develop on skin tending to be seborrhoeic, affect mainly the face and produce papules and pustules. Rosacea most commonly develops in adulthood, between the 40th and 50th years of life. It begins with redness in the central parts of the face — nose, middle of forehead, cheek areas near the nose. The redness appears particularly when temperatures get warmer — moving from a cool to a warm room, drinking something hot, exposure to the sun and consumption of alcohol (skin vessels expand, increasing blood supply). Small red veins then also appear in the reddened areas, and later also papules and pustules. The pus in the pustules characteristically does not contain bacteria. As with acne, the condition arises from the sebaceous glands; but rosacea does not involve increased numbers of blackheads. Rosacea may persist for decades and gradually cause the tissues of the nose to grow coarse and enlarged (bulbous nose, rhinophyma), though this happens only to men.

A constitutional tendency towards increased sebum flow and the presence of more blood in the skin and even inflammation of the sebaceous glands in the lower dermis point to excessive metabolism. Metabolic processes are too powerful, going beyond the norm. The centre of metabolism lies below the diaphragm. If metabolic activity gets excessive in the skin of the face, the thought comes to mind that there has been a shift upwards, beyond the boundary set by the diaphragm, and that metabolic organs in the abdomen have slowed down in their functions. It is not uncommon to find disorders affecting liver and gall bladder, stomach and intestine in people suffering from rosacea. Alcohol may play a role in putting a strain on the liver, but this need not be the case.

The treatment of rosacea must take these things into account. If there are signs of problems in the epigastric (upper abdominal) organs, medical treatment is needed to activate metabolism (P). Homoeopathic medicines restrain the blood from pushing too much up into the facial skin. Antimony has the powers needed for this, for example (P). Externally, drying suspensions containing sulphur are used (P). Massaging in Dr Hauschka Rhythmic Conditioner, Sensitive, at night, will calm the situation in the skin (S).

Perioral dermatitis (inflammatory lesions around the mouth)

Perioral dermatitis is the term used for a condition seen mainly in young women between the ages of 20 and 30. It has become more widespread in recent decades, like an epidemic. The skin is reddened and scaly, with tiny lesions, mostly around the mouth, the sides of the nose and in the nasolabial fold (fold running from nose to lips). The small red lesions may also appear on the lower lid. Moisturizing creams are often the cause of the problem, which does affect cosmetic appearance. They may have been well tolerated for years of daily use, but then the point comes where the skin has clearly grown tired of this 'good' treatment and will no longer tolerate the usual care. Inappropriate local use of corticosteroids may also be a cause. Digestive weakness is less often indicated as a possible cause of this skin disorder.

As the cause is generally external, we must also deal with the situation from outside. Omit the moisturizing cream and use a suspension or ointment containing zinc oxide (S). If the skin needs replenishing during the day, Almond Intensive Facial Cream[1] is usually well tolerated (S). Dr Hauschka Toned Day Cream is also suitable (S); it soothes the skin irritation. If the skin is much reddened or actually weeping, compresses of cold St John's wort tea are very effective (S). If the condition proves resistant, an ointment containing an antibiotic will help to heal it (P).

Granuloma annulare

The Latin term means 'ring-shaped lesion'. The condition is quite common and completely benign. The lesions appear most often on the extensor (outside) sides of hands and feet and near the ankles. They arise from the dermis, with the epidermis quite unaffected. The lesions often merge into rings and show a tendency to spread centrifugally whilst healing at the centre. They cause no symptoms and often heal spontaneously within two years.

Granuloma annulare usually has no evident triggers. Suggested causes have been insect bites, skin injuries, infections and diabetes, but this is doubtful. Children and young people are mostly affected, and females twice as often as males, which establishes certain characteristics for the condition. The growing organism and the female constitution, which is more closely connected to powers of growth, evidently provide the right soil for this skin problem. Granuloma annulare is therefore due to overweening powers of growth. These create dense nodules in the matrix of the dermis and make it swell.

Sometimes just taking a sample of the skin (for study under the microscope), thus causing a minor injury, may be all it needs to induce healing. Or fine scratches across the lesions, making them bleed just a little, may also do the trick (P). The lesions often heal if you simply cover them with a sticking plaster (S). It is worth trying Antimonite 0.4% Ointment[1], a thin layer massaged into the skin over the lesions once a day for some weeks (S).

Urticaria (nettle rash)

Nettle rash owes its name to the hives or wheals which look as if one had touched a stinging nettle (*Urtica*). The hives range in size from a penny to the palm of a hand, are reddened and slightly raised. The itching is often terrible. The lesions may appear as an eruption all over the body. They are due to the expansion of fine blood vessels in the upper dermis; this causes the redness. Blood serum oozing from the vessels (extravasation) makes the upper dermis swell up, hence the characteristic raised form of hives. The extravasation may go so far that increasing pressure in the tissues expresses the blood from the vessels; the hives then grow as pale as porcelain. The site of vessel expansion and extravasation may, however, also be deeper down in the skin. The fatty tissues in the subcutis then fill up, so that the whole of an upper arm may swell up like dough (angio-oedema). Such deep-seated

101

swelling in the regions of the lips and mucous membrane lining the mouth and throat as well as in the tongue is called angioneurotic oedema; it may block the upper respiratory tract and then be life-threatening.

An acute bout of urticaria may involve dyspnoea (difficulty breathing) and circulatory problems. Dyspnoea is due to spasm in the bronchial musculature, with tough mucus developing, as with asthma. The circulation is affected by a drop in blood pressure as blood is withdrawn from the skin and head (fainting) in a state of shock. In this case, the cause is usually an allergic reaction.

Compared to allergic contact dermatitis (late-type allergy), where sensitized defence cells cause the skin inflammation, specific antibodies, immunoglobulins E, play a role in urticaria. A substance – perhaps a medicine such as an analgesic – is taken into the blood via the intestine and stimulates the production of an immunoglobulin specialized in fighting that substance. In most cases the medicine has been no problem though taken for years. Suddenly sensitization develops, the medicine becomes an allergen and the organism produces an allergic reaction to it with the specific antibodies.

The process is often helped by the organism being weakened following an infection or due to stress. Once sensitization has occurred and the specific antibodies exist, the allergic reaction takes only minutes to appear. This is therefore called an instant-type allergy. It is the basis of allergic urticaria, allergic asthma, hay fever with conjunctivitis, and allergic shock.

Checking if someone is allergic to a specific substance may be done in two ways. Laboratory tests can determine the specific antibodies in the blood. A skin test is more informative, however. Apply one drop of a solution containing the allergen in question in a specific concentration and prick the skin through that drop, using a special needle. If the person is allergic to the substance, the skin will react soon after this, raising a weal. The test can be 'read' after 20 minutes.

The causes of urticaria are many. It may be an allergy, as shown above, or the immune system may not be involved at all; in that case one speaks of a pseudoallergy. The distinction cannot be made by looking at the nettle rash from outside.

Nettle rash can be triggered by:

- foods — fish, seafood, some blue cheeses, strawberries, gooseberries, walnuts, citrus fruit, pulses, tomatoes, celery or celeriac
- herbs or spices (e.g. dill)
- coffee, drinks containing quinine, some wines
- intestinal worms, intestinal yeast infections
- viral infections
- bee's venom, wasp venom
- medicines — most often painkillers
- vaccines

It is important for people suffering from urticaria to know those triggers, for the physician can only find the causes if he knows the patient's observations. It can be helpful to keep a diary to try and establish the connection between urticaria and foods, spices, stimulants such as coffee, or medicines.

Other triggers may be heat, cold and external pressure. There is also one kind which arises due to physical overexertion. The condition may also accompany diseases such as rheumatic conditions. Weals that rise under every close-fitting garment and every time the skin is scratched are particularly unpleasant. In this case, a mark made on the skin with a blunt fingernail will raise a weal within a few minutes. This type of urticaria points to autonomic instability, often confirmed when the physician takes a closer look.

None of the above-mentioned triggers may be found in a large proportion of people with urticaria. Extensive statistical analyses have shown, however, that in most of them the autonomic nervous system is easily excited and there is a tendency to be nervous, anxious and suffer from mood changes. Stress can be a trigger in this case, often coming from the social environment. These are psychological problems involving powerful mental reactions and emotions, and it is easy to make the individual concerned aware of this. Social conflicts will easily enrage, cause anxiety or feelings of powerlessness and hopelessness. Great joy can also trigger a bout of nettle rash. Looking at the situation from outside, one gains the impression that these individuals go from one extreme to another in their mind and feelings, like a rudderless skiff on the mighty billows of the open sea.

In this case treatment will consist in the physician helping the patient to be aware of situations where a bout of weals is triggered via the psyche. Self-knowledge makes it possible to take the helm again and guide the skiff into calmer waters. As time goes on, such self-knowledge will establish more calm in the emotional life. Over-excitability of the autonomic nervous system can be counteracted with hot and cold contrast baths, Kneipp treatments and physical exercise.

If food triggers have been established (e.g. fish), or there are gastrointestinal disorders (e.g. yeast infection of the intestine), digestive powers must be strengthened with herbal and homoeopathic medicines (P). In severe cases, progress will only be made following a mild derivative diet after F. X. Mayr (P). This includes laxative treatment with bitter salt and nettle tea as well as horsetail tea (P).

A whole range of medicines based on minerals and plants are also available, examples being calcium, oak bark, tin and stinging nettle (*Urtica urens*) (P). Recommended self-medication includes Calcium carbonicum/Cortex quercus Pilules[2], 10 pilules 2–5 times a day before meals, or Urtica comp. Globuli[2], 10 pilules 1–3 times a day before meals (S). Dermatodoron[1] is suitable (P) for treating urticaria due to cold temperatures.

Pruritus, burning pain and sensations of heat will usually respond immediately in a bout of nettle rash if Combudoron Gel[1] or Wund- und Brandgel (soothing gel)[2] is applied thinly over whole skin areas several times a day (S). Compresses of Combudoron Lotion[1] (diluted 1 : 10 in water) or Brandessenz (essence of Urtica)[2] (1 tablespoon to 250 ml of water) are even more cooling (S); both of these must not be used by anyone who is allergic to arnica.

Hay fever

Everyone knows about hay fever today, a very common condition in western industrialized countries. It is not a skin disease in the narrower sense but will be considered here because it does quite often occur together with neurodermatitis, and dermatologists have to treat the two conditions together. It is also almost always due to an allergy, and can teach us a great deal about allergic reactions.

Mild hay fever merely means a blocked nose, so that one has to breathe through the mouth and the person concerned tends to snore at night. Taste and smell are often affected or even lost altogether. With more severe forms, the nose is running, and the secretion is always clear. Secretions turn yellow or even greenish if they contain pus, which suggests a cold caused by bacteria. The nerves in the nasal mucosa (lining) are irritated and the person sneezes, often producing a whole string of sneezes (sneezing attack). If the mucous membranes of the eyes are affected as well, the eyes will itch and water, and the person concerned tends to rub them. Swelling of the mucous membranes means that fluid is collecting; this fluid binds powers that should really be available for wide-awake thinking. People with hay fever therefore often feel hazy; they find it difficult to concentrate when their hay fever is in full spate.

In children, hay fever is more governed by metabolism. The constitutional background is often one of lively activity in the senses, with the soul drawn to the periphery. This has two consequences. 1) The child grows hypersensitive in the sphere of the senses; he takes in too much and tends to overreact. 2) With the soul's involvement shifted to the sphere of the senses from its middle position between above and below, inside and outside, there is not enough soul activity in the inner organism, e.g. in the digestion. Food is not properly broken down as digestive juices lack bite, and the child's organism is flooded with half-digested matter to which the life of the food plant and the foreign soul qualities of the animal (for meat eaters) still adhere. Those foreign substances act like poisons and must be eliminated; the necessary elimination then goes via the allergic reaction in the mucous membranes.

In adults, the causes of hay fever are best seen if we take a closer look at springtime hay fever. In winter, people living in the temperate zones are more inward in their psyche, being able, for instance, to enter into Christmas as something that happens wholly in the soul. In spring, the ascending sun gains in strength and stimulates life in the plant and animal worlds; the earth exhales its powers. Human beings also exhale at the level of the psyche as they enter into the joys of spring and delight in the natural world. People who constitutionally tend to have the emphasis on the neurosensory system are then in particular danger of exhaling too strongly in the psyche, with the soul coming loose from the basis of the living physical body. The human soul lives in the airy element in the organism;

everything watery and solid is fully formed out, given powers of form, by the airy principle. If the soul has loosened, this weakens the powers of form coming from the airy principle, and the water organism brings its formless laws to bear, that is, the mucous membranes swell up. If the soul is too active in the sense organs, this leads to hypersensitivity; the water organism wants to 'extinguish' this but overshoots the mark and 'drowns' the area where this is going on. The mucous membranes swell up as a result.

The tendency is in our time to ascribe all illness to external factors and physical substances. A long list of external triggers is therefore known to allergologists. Grass pollen heads the list, having given hay fever its name, for in the past hay was made at times when the grass was flowering. Grass flowers contain much pollen and long, thin but strong stems keep them at a relatively great distance from the vegetative region where the leaves are down below. The pollen, being dry and extremely light, tends to spread widely through the surroundings. (Grasses are wind-pollinated.) We might compare it to a gas which, once released, wants to mingle with the air in the atmosphere. Every pollen grain has a finely worked, differentiated surface which differs from one species to another, evidence that powers of form from the cosmic periphery are intensely involved. It is those powers of form (or rather the work they have done) which prove such an irritant to the hypersensitive individual with hay fever.

Apart from grass pollen, hay fever is often caused by pollen from early flowering trees, and also by dust mites, animal hairs (dogs, cats, horses, rabbits) and feathers. Physical factors such as light, heat, cold and dust can also provoke the symptoms. The prick test may be used to confirm the diagnosis, but in most cases reliable information on the triggers involved comes directly from the pattern of the condition (all the year round or connected with a particular season, morning or

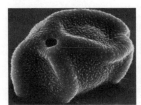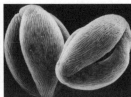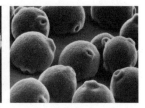

Pollen from alder, maple and birch seen under the scanning electron microscope

evening/night, indoors or outdoors, contact with particular animals, visits to particular places).

Generally speaking, people who are able to give themselves up to the beauties of nature and to go dreamy in spring are less likely to have hay fever than someone who is nervous or anxious about creepy-crawlies and things blowing in the wind.

The aim in treating hay fever to achieve a genuine cure must be to bring the extra water which has gathered in the mucous membranes of nose and eyes under control. Centrifugal forces have made the nasal mucosa as watery as the mucosa of the small intestine. Lemon (*Citrus medica*) and quince (*Cydonia oblonga*) act in the opposite, centripetal direction, being astringent. The leathery skin of both defines the fruit well against the environment. The taste of these fruits also tells us much. It makes the mouth pucker up, in the case of lemon because it is acid, in that of quince due to tartness. Gencydo[1] and Citrus/Cydonia[2] are medicines containing extracts from both. For adults, they are best given by subcutaneous injection (P), which causes a slight burning sensation. We have a parallel here to the effect which draws the soul element together again so that it may take hold of the living physical body. The injections are most effective if given above the seventh cervical vertebra (this projects slightly when the head is bent forwards and can be felt to project). This site is exactly opposite to the nose on the other side of the head, where the problem has arisen. A simple image will illustrate the effect of this treatment. Two little boys are standing at an open window on the fourth floor of a house and want to see who can bend furthest forward. Their mother will be horrified when she sees this and grabs them by the collar to yank them back into the room. This is how it is when soul activities reach out too far through the gates of the senses. Gencydo or Citrus/Cydonia fetches them back into the organism.

Gencydo is also available as an ointment to apply to the inside of the nose, as Gencydo solution for instilling into the nose (S), and Gencydo Eye Drops (P). The effect of Gencydo and Citrus/Cydonia is best if injections are started a month before the season begins – twice a week, using the lowest concentration. It is not uncommon for symptoms to get less from year to year or disappear altogether, so that there will then be no need for further treatment.

Gencydo and Citrus/Cydonia are the main medicines used in

anthroposophical medical hay fever treatment. The action is deep-reaching, and they will be effective with any allergy that produces hay fever. It is therefore not necessary to know the allergen responsible and there is no need for a prick test. A further possibility is to treat functional weakness of the liver, which is the central organ in the fluid organism. Poor regulation of this function can provide the basis for hay fever. Tin (Stannum) in potentized form has a harmonizing effect on the watery principle (P). Much the same applies to potassium carbonate in potentized form (P).

Desensitization or hyposensitization plays a major role in the conventional treatment of allergies and will often prove highly effective. In this case, exact knowledge of the allergen is essential, that is, a prick test must always be done. The allergen or a combination of allergens is then injected subcutaneously in slowly rising doses at intervals of some days. This gradually gets the organism used to the allergen, a slightly sneaky way of getting rid of the sensitization. The method does not, of course, go more deeply into the constitutional background of the hay fever which also needs to be dealt with. Desensitization also costs time and money, and there is a residual risk of severe general allergic reactions which may prove fatal if an overdose is given by mistake.

Sunlight sensitivity (allergy to sunlight)

When the sunlight grows more intense in the spring or on holiday in the sunny south in winter, young women will often develop an eruption which is caused by the UV part of it. The eruption may take very different forms in different people – red spots, weals, small nodular lesions, all of them usually very itchy. They are therefore also called 'polymorphic [many forms] light eruptions'. The signs are, however, the same year after year in one and the same person. The eruptions appear in all areas that have been exposed to the sun – face, arms, back of the hands, neckline area. They disappear as soon as the sun is avoided. The organism gets used to the sun during the summer, and allergy to sunlight occurs only in March to June in our latitudes.

It is assumed that specific proteins in the blood in the skin undergo a change on exposure to sun to trigger the eruption. This suggests metabolic abnormalities. Phototoxic and photoallergic dermatitis may also be part of the background to sunlight allergy.

One external cause is the fact that people are travelling a lot more, going to the sunny south also in the winter months. At the same time, the quality of sunlight has changed. The ozone layer is now known to have grown thinner not only over the South Pole but also over the northern hemisphere. This means that more of the UV part of sunlight reaches the earth's surface. Older people who have been working on farms all their lives know from experience that the sun's rays are more aggressive today than they were in the past.

Externally, protection against sunlight involves using the sunscreen products manufactured by Weleda and Wala, for example, covering up well, and letting the skin get used to the sun gradually as the intensity of its rays increases in spring. Taking carrots or carrot juice daily with a little cream (carotene is fat-soluble and the organism cannot take it up unless fat is present) will give the skin a slightly yellowy-brown colouring and make it resistant to the sun (S). St John's wort provides excellent prevention. Take drops of a homoeopathic preparation of it in relatively high dilution (P). If an eruption has developed, Combu-doron products[1], Wund- und Brandgel (soothing gel)[2] or a zinc sus-pension (S) will give relief (S). Internally, one may take Urtica comp. Pilules[2], 10 pilules 1–3 times a day before meals (S).

Alopecia (hair loss)

The transition from hair loss as a variable within healthy limits to an actual disorder is a gradual one. Roughly speaking, the loss of up to 100 hairs a day is normal. It also depends on how much new hair is growing. Mild or severe and therefore pathological hair loss occurs for a variety of reasons, which are briefly listed below:

- disorders in the digestive tract resulting in nutritional problems for hair
- functional liver disorders
- anaemia and iron deficiency
- medicines, e.g. heparin to prevent thrombosis
- hormonal changes, e.g. due to pregnancy, the pill or the menopause
- following infectious diseases such as hepatitis

- inflammatory changes in the scalp, e.g. seborrhoeic dermatitis, psoriasis
- male-type hair loss
- seasonal or climatic changes in spring and autumn

Brief mention was made, on pages 6–7, of the 28-day moon rhythm in the vital processes of the epidermis. Hair has its roots in the lower dermis, but the roots are an appendage of the epidermis extending down into the depths of the dermis. Hair growth is also influenced by the moon. It is stimulated if hair is cut just before full moon, ideally with the moon in Leo. (For an exact moon calendar, see Maria Thun's *Biodynamic Sowing & Planting Calendar*.) All it needs is to cut off a few millimetres. In earlier times, the time for visiting a barber was carefully chosen. A silver disk hanging outside the shop indicated the days when the moon was in the right position for a haircut to stimulate growth.

It is also recommended to massage Rosemary Hair Lotion[1] or Neem Hair Lotion[2] into the scalp daily (S). Wash hair once a week to

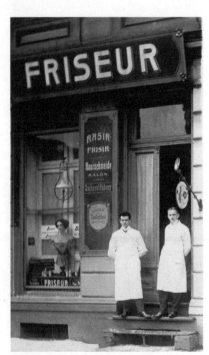

'nourish', using a mixture of 1 teaspoonful of castor oil and 1 egg yolk (S). Wet the hair thoroughly before massaging in the mixture. Leave to act for 20 minutes, then rinse repeatedly in tepid chamomile tea. If this is too cumbersome, use Dr Hauschka Neem Oil applications which also nourish the hair and scalp (S). Massage a few drops into the wet scalp and leave for 20 minutes before shampooing. Nettle tea also stimulates hair growth. Pour a litre of boiling water on 2 tablespoons of the dried leaves (chopped fresh leaves in spring), leave to stand for 3 minutes (only $\frac{1}{2}$ minute for fresh leaves), then strain through a sieve. Take the first cup on an empty stomach in the morning,

Historical photograph of silver disc outside barber's shop

and divide the rest over the day. Do this for six to eight weeks. Barley and millet provide the organism with silica for hair growth; it is recommended to have both of them at least once a week, instead of potatoes at the main meal, for instance. Generally speaking, a balanced wholefood diet provides a sound basis for hair growth. These, then, are the general measures that make for healthy hair.

The causes listed above for different organic regions will, of course, need specialist treatment. A digestive disorder must be treated with anthroposophical medicines, as the stream of constructive substance in the blood starts from the thorough breaking down of food in the digestive tract and extends as far as feeding the live root of a hair (P). If liver function is sluggish, treatment to vitalize the liver will show results also in the vitality of the hair root (P). Iron gives impulses and form to anabolism. If the organism's ability to take hold of iron in the food and metabolize it is failing, stinging nettle is one of the medicinal agents which can stimulate that function (P).

Finally, reference should also be made to male-pattern baldness, for which there is no remedy.

It occurs in women as well, with hair growing thin over the temples and in the middle part of the scalp. One could try and stimulate the function of the ovaries, which would change the relative proportions of hormones in favour of female ones (P).

Patchy hair loss (alopecia areata)

In one particular form of hair loss the immune system suddenly turns against the body's own tissues, in this case the hair roots. A small area of inflammation develops around the root in the lower dermis, and the hair is lost. This usually happens in coin-sized circular areas. Many such areas may develop and also join up; if the condition is extensive this affects not only the scalp but also the eyebrows and the beard area. In the worst case, all hair will be lost. Alopecia areata is more common in children, but may also develop in adults. Serious worries will quite often trigger it, or biographical crises, for instance the death of a close relative. This casts some light on the underlying causes. The interplay between anabolism and catabolism in the skin, between life and death, shifts towards the side of death even to the point where the hair dies.

This also gives the direction which treatment should take. To counteract the destructive nervous processes and defensive processes directed against the individual's own hair, we must direct the constructive bloodstream to the skin. This can be done by exposure to sun until the skin reddens slightly or by using ointments designed to treat rheumatic conditions (e.g. Finalgon, manuf. by Boehringer) that encourage blood circulation and the generation of heat (P). A gentle alternative to Finalgon is Cera/Aesculus comp. Ointment[2] (S). A dermatologist will use UV radiation in his practice, perhaps in combination with light-sensitizing substances. Another method is to use chemicals that provoke allergy in anyone to produce a mild skin eruption. This diverts the inflammatory process from the bulb of the hair root in the lower dermis to the upper dermis and epidermis. This treatment is still in the process of development, however, and only done in the outpatient departments of dermatological clinics. A gentler method of treatment is the daily application of a hair lotion containing essential oil of rosemary 10% and Arnica Essence 50%[1] in alcohol (S). A whole range of potentized medicines is also available (P).

Vitiligo

The immune system can turn not only against hair roots, as with patchy hair loss, but also against the pigment-producers in the epidermis, interfering with pigment production or killing those particular cells. Physical stress may be a trigger, e.g. due to sunburn, or mental stress at work or at home. Depigmented areas often appear first in the face, on the neck and hands; they increase slowly in size and may also extend to other areas.

Treatment is not easy. If the white areas are less than two years old, anthroposophical medical treatment (P) may be effective.

Scleroderma (systemic sclerosis)

Scleroderma literally means 'hardened skin' in Latin. It is a connective tissue disease affecting the skin and internal organs, an autoimmune disease where the immune system turns its proteins and defence cells against the body's own tissues, causing them to grow inflamed. Initially the skin therefore shows swelling; then skin and subcutis harden and finally tighten up.

A circumscribed, focal form of scleroderma affects the skin only. The foci are red at first, then harden, and finally form slight, scarlike depressions. Inflammation in a coin-sized focus will often spread centrifugally, producing a characteristic picture. At the centre of the focus is a yellowy, pale, hard plaque, firmly adherent to the tissues under the skin; it has a reddish-violet ring around it.

Another form of scleroderma is extensive, affecting the whole skin, with the emphasis often on face and hands. The patient will be highly sensitive to cold in the cold season of the year; hands and feet, and also nose and ears, are cold and a reddish blue. There may be episodes when individual fingers turn white and cold, look dead and are painful as if gone to sleep. This is due to spasms in the fine arteries. Hardening of the skin is first apparent in the cuticles in the nail fold; these grow cornified, bleed and tear. The fingers grow thin and rigid and can no longer be fully stretched and bent. Hardening of the skin is also evident in the face. Facial expression is limited in its mobility, the face grows smaller, and radial folds develop around the mouth. The skin condition may (but need not) be accompanied by similar connective tissue hardening in internal organs – the digestive tract, lungs and kidneys.

The character of scleroderma is determined by the irreversible outcome of the inflammation – hardening, reduced circulation, loss of heat, life receding in the tissues, and tissue loss. The inflammatory stage with redness and swelling is an attempt at self-healing. Ultimately, however, the excessive form principle keeps the upper hand. The causes of scleroderma are not known in conventional medicine.

The simplest way of supporting the weakened warmth organism is to keep warm by wearing warm clothes, shoes and gloves. Smokers must stop smoking altogether, for nicotine supports loss of heat from the body periphery. Baths with the stimulating essential oil of rosemary or soothing, relaxing lavender (use Weleda or Wala bath products) can be recommended (S). The essential oils contained in them have developed in the hot sun of the Mediterranean and are heat turned into matter. They stimulate the warmth organism and thus also the human I which is active within it. The I itself cannot fall ill; it is the driving force in all self-healing. With scleroderma it counterbalances excessive powers of form with powers of matter, reducing them to a healthy level. Reference was made to oil dispersion baths in the section on neurodermatitis. These are also very suitable for scleroderma (S). Good oils for this are Rosemary Oil 10%[2] and Lavender Oil 10%[2].

Medical treatment is with mistletoe preparations, which are injected under the skin (P). Red ant (Formica) by subcutaneous injection or taken in form of drops helps to dissolve the hardening (P). Lead sulphide (galenite), injected under the skin in relatively high potencies, will also help to control the tendency to harden (P).

Pigmented moles (naevi, birthmarks)

Pigmented moles may develop anywhere on the skin in variable numbers and sizes immediately after birth, or may be present even at birth. New moles may be added until about the middle of life, the 35th year. It is not uncommon for them to resolve at a more advanced age. They may be dots, patches, the size of a palm or even larger. Smallish moles are flat or raised like warts. Really large ones, often very dark, with warty surface and quite a few hairs, tend to degenerate more often than the small ones do, and should therefore be inspected annually by a specialist.

The cells that produce the brown pigment in the skin are normally evenly 'scattered' in the lower layer of the epidermis. A mole develops where they stop being solitary and gather in groups; they 'clot'. They may then also leave the epidermis and settle in the neighbouring upper dermis.

It depends primarily on heredity whether someone has many moles, just a few or none at all. The condition generally runs in families. It may also happen, however, that the disposition to have many moles is not inherited from the parents but comes entirely on its own.

It is interesting to note that the number of moles also depends on the number of times someone has had sunburn in childhood. It is now known that every sunburn before the age of 20 will result in more moles; this is no longer the case after the age of 20. It tells us something about the nature of moles when they appear in great numbers in someone. Sunlight, the main representative of sensory stimuli, can interfere with the regular distribution of pigment pro-ducers. If its intensity leads to sunburn, this clearly stresses the skin and throws the 'sunscreen' in the epidermis into disorder. The pig-ment producers 'clot together'. Think of bits of gravel on a tray thrown into confusion if you knock against the tray. Sunburn would be one possible way in which moles may develop, though not every mole. Other causes have not become known in conventional science, however.

Not everyone has noticeable moles, and not everyone has many moles. Some people who were certainly exposed to the sun a great deal in childhood still do not have many moles. So who does develop them? What do these marks on the skin signify for the whole person? If as a dermatologist you reflect on a large number of people who have many moles, it may strike you that many among them are quite generally sensitive to environmental stimuli. All the many different impressions flooding in from all directions cannot always be coped with as a matter of course, however many they may be. It needs strength to cope with them. Perhaps it is important for people with many moles to know that they are among the more sen-sitive individuals and need to accept that they have this disposition, and take note of all the things that influence them and of what they must do to 'digest' them properly.

Protection from too much sun – this is what the dermatologist must advise for people with many moles. (See the section on Melanoma, pages 119–27, for details of the changes which sunlight can cause in moles, ranging from chaos in the structure of the mole to degeneration into cancer.) It would be fair, I think, to extend the need for protection shown by people with many moles to all external influences. They should not take on too much work and responsibility both at home and at work.

Port-wine stain (naevus flammeus) and strawberry marks (haemangioma)

These blueish red to bright red, flat marks are usually present from birth. In the newborn one often sees them near the hairline on the head or at the back of the neck. The latter are also known as 'stork bites', the

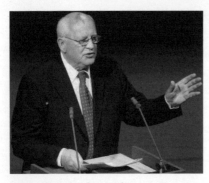

Michail Gorbachev with port-wine stain on forehead

idea being that the stork bringing the baby had to hold him in its beak at that point. The rapid rise of former Russian President Gorbachev made him widely known, and also the port-wine stain on his forehead. Such stains develop as small blood vessels in the upper dermis widen and increase in numbers. The condition is benign. Removal is possible using a high-tech laser.

If the increase in blood vessels produces a bluish red raised area, this is known as a strawberry mark (haemangioma). Such lesions develop weeks or months after birth and are mostly located on the head, though they may also occur in any other location. They are always benign and usually disappear again completely or almost completely. A strawberry mark can be very disfiguring, for instance if it appears beside the nose. Parents are advised to be patient and wait for it to disappear. Any residues can be removed later with a laser. It is possible to try and influence this dynamic process of the birthmark developing and fading away with anthroposophical medicines (P). Antimonite 0.4% Ointment or Stibium metallicum prep. 0.4% Ointment[1], applied thinly twice a day to the mark lets powers of form radiate into the excessive vascular development (S).

The skin of older people will often show brilliant red marks the size of a grain of rice. These are completely benign and just a sign of getting older. They can be removed with electrically generated heat if desired for cosmetic reasons.

Warts of old age (seborrhoeic keratosis)

Wartlike thickened patches are more commonly seen in the second half of life. They are usually one half to one centimetre in diameter, greyish brown, light to dark brown or even black and may appear in considerable numbers in old people. Most appear on the trunk and face, in skin areas with many sebaceous glands – hence the term 'seborrhoeic warts'. They do not degenerate. It is difficult for lay people to differentiate them from malignant skin lesions. It is advisable to have a skin specialist inspect the 'crop' from time to time.

If one would like to be rid of such a wart for cosmetic reasons, this is easily done by an expert using a scalpel.

Age spots (lentigines)

Age spots are more or less brown, flat spots appearing mainly in skin areas much exposed to sunlight – face, outside of forearms and back of hands. They occur in the second half of life. The term lentigo (plural 'lentigines') comes from the Latin for lentil, as they often are lentil-size. They are produced by exposure to the sun and will never degenerate.

It is possible to bleach lentigines, but the effect will not last. It is also possible to remove them with cryotherapy or a laser.

The ageing skin

Under the microscope, the skin of an old person shows a thinner epidermis, with papillae in the upper dermis grown flatter, and the whole dermis containing fewer connective tissue fibres. This also makes the dermis thinner. The subcutis contains less fat. We may thus speak of shrinkage (involution) affecting all layers in the skin of old people. Blood circulation gets less, as does the water content; the skin loses elasticity. Sebaceous and sweat glands are less productive. In old age the whole organism gradually becomes less vital, and anabolism in the skin is also reduced. Blood vessels grow fragile, and bruises may develop even from slight bumps.

The visible outcome of all those processes is a skin that is a bit too big, flaccid, easily creased and vulnerable. Large blood vessels show through. The most marked indication of ageing is the growing number of wrinkles. Ageing and the development of wrinkles are above all encouraged by sunlight. The more sun has reached the skin in the course of life, the thinner and more wrinkled will it be in old age. This applies especially to uncovered skin areas – face, back of neck, backs of hands and forearms. Much exposure to the sun leaves more of a mark in fair-haired and light-skinned people than in dark skin types. Fair-complexioned people develop wrinkles much faster in the south. Ageing in the skin is also accelerated if the skin is not properly nourished, in times of starvation, for instance, or due to illness (e.g. a liver disease). Serious worries also make the skin age faster, and the menopause often involves a phase where a woman's skin ages more quickly.

Dryness is another indication that metabolic functions in the skin are decreasing. Dermatitis can quickly develop (see section on Dermatitis in the elderly, pages 92–93). Hardening tendencies increase throughout the organism in old age, with the skin growing cornified lesions due to the influence of light (actinic keratosis), usually over a red spot. These are precursors of skin cancer developing from horn cells (see section on Squamous cell carcinoma, pages 128–129). They need to have an eye kept on them, and if they bleed or fail to heal up after a weeping stage, a dermatologist must be consulted.

Many things in western civilization make us attach considerably more importance to the first half of life, when we build up our physical body, to the outer aspects of existence and to social life than we do to the second half of life with its processes of involution (physical regression). Growing physical frailty and death are banished from the mind in a way of thinking that concentrates on material life. We can therefore understand why so much effort is put into using cosmetics to hide the ageing skin today.

In physiology, the law applies that destruction and involution go hand in hand with an increase in processes that lead to conscious awareness (and vice versa). This means that the ageing skin and wrinkles must be seen in a different light. Ageing at the organic level is connected with a broadening of mental horizons, wisdom of life gained. (The fact that this is not automatically the case with everyone does not disprove it.) Why don't we have a go at adopting this view? Why don't we learn to appreciate the lines in the face of someone who is growing older?

The most formed out and individual skin area is the face, with differentiated muscles permitting facial expression. When we contract a facial muscle, the skin is pushed together in that place. Laughter lines, lines of care, and so on develop as a result, running at right angles to the muscles. This is how a person's individual nature is reflected in the face, and also in its lines. The pleasures and pain of a life leave their mark; events in the biography give the face its character. The connection between one particular kind of inner nature and its outer physical form can be studied really well in Native North Americans. You'll need to look at nineteenth-century photographs, however, to see what I mean. Bony, slender, angular body form, a solemn, much-lined face go together with the wisdom of the most ancient Native American spirituality relating to the natural world. This is no longer so evident in the faces of Native North Americans today, for the modern American lifestyle is all too often connected with obesity.

Cosmetic efforts to cover up the fact that skin is ageing may thus be looked at with a critical eye. I advise against the external and internal use of female hormones. It is possible and has not so far been disproved that breast cancer is encouraged when oestrogens are taken after the menopause. It also makes the process of maturing in the psyche difficult if not impossible. Outwardly this shows in a keenness on competitive sports that is not appropriate to that age and a refusal to entertain thoughts concerning the time limits set to all life on earth.

Ageing skin needs regular care to provide it with fats. Use soap as little as possible, shower or take a bath once a week at most. Permanent use of a cream with a moderate degree of sunscreen factor on all skin areas exposed to light is recommended, such as the Weleda sunscreen products which contain an extract of edelweiss, and Dr Hauschka sunscreen products (titanium dioxide, zinc oxide). Old skin damaged by light may be treated with Birch Cream (manuf. by Birken GmbH); the extract of birch cork it contains can repair such damage. The base of it is just avocado and almond oil; this means that allergic reactions to Birch Cream are practically nil, making it suitable for daily use. For details of Dr Hauschka-trained stockists and aestheticians in your area contact the address given at the back of this book. Echinacea/Viscum comp. Gel[2], which is fat-free, vitalizes the skin quite generally. The right diet for old age has effects that extend also to the skin. Fruits that store honey and water, such as melon, are particularly suitable. Milk, with its powerful anabolic effects should be taken in moderation.

Melanoma (malignant melanoma)

Melanoma develops when the pigment producers (melanocytes) in the lower epidermis degenerate and become cancerous. Some melanomas are initially a dark spot which develops as cells increase and spread horizontally, without crossing the boundary to the dermis. Years may pass at this stage. Later, melanoma cells migrate into the dermis and possibly also into blood and lymph vessels. Another, smaller proportion of melanomas will immediately grow vertically downwards. Healthy melanocytes exist in isolation in the skin and are mobile. This mobility persists also for melanoma cells, and this makes the condition malignant. It is not uncommon for metastases (satellite tumours) to develop in the lymph nodes for the affected skin region and/or via the blood in internal organs.

Melanomas develop mostly in the middle of life. Women have them mainly in the face and on the legs, men more often on the upper trunk. Some melanomas develop on normal skin, others on pre-existing pigmented moles.

How does a skin specialist assess the risk of melanoma in looking at someone's skin? In order of importance, the indications are as follows:

- number of pigmented moles
- number of pigmented moles showing irregular form
- number of age spots due to exposure to sun
- fair hair and fair skin type.

We will go into these in more detail below. With regard to aggressiveness at different age levels, melanoma is like many other forms of cancer. The older the patient, the slower the growth, that is, the more benign the melanoma.

The incidence of melanoma is on the increase the world over. In central Europe, the number of new melanomas was found to have doubled in ten years. What makes this type of tumour occur more often? What does melanoma have to do with people of today?

Generally speaking the increase in melanoma is ascribed to changed ways of spending leisure time and therefore increased exposure to the sun. This is no doubt one of the causes; but it does not apply to all the melanoma patients who were careful about exposure to the sun all their lives, being light sensitive. To come closer to finding an answer to the above questions, let us take a look at two groups of people – those with many moles and those with fair skin.

Someone with about 50 or more pigmented moles may be said to have many. The special traits in body and soul of people with pigmented moles have been considered in that section above (pages 114–15). Sunburn in childhood (up to the age of 20) increases the number and therefore the melanoma risk. It is interesting to note that the number of pigmented moles with irregular structure increases in line with the number of sunburn episodes. The irregularities can be seen with the naked eye; some of the characteristics are:

- irregular pigmentation, piebald appearance, pale brown and black parts
- lack of symmetry, that is, not round or oval but bizarre forms
- irregular borders, sometimes clearly defined, other times not
- diameter of more than 5 mm.

These changes in the architecture of a mole are also apparent under the microscope. A dermatologist will therefore take a closer look at skin showing many moles and search for those that appear atypical in form. Both a large number of moles and the atypical moles may be signs that the skin, and hence the boundaries in body and soul, are under particular stress.

If fair-haired people of light skin type tend to develop melanoma more than people with dark hair and skin, the question is: Where does the difference lie in people who have such different capacities for pigmentation? Those with great 'impulse power' in the nutrient blood push nutrients all the way to the eye, the hair and skin; they have brown eyes, black hair and dark skin. The blackness of earth is driven powerfully to the periphery of the organism.

Blue-eyed people with fair hair and skin have less impulse power in the blood. Pigment producers have the same density in their skin as in people of the dark type, but they are not as productive, producing less brown pigment. In this particular respect people with fair hair and skin are therefore weaker in body, and this is hereditary. On the other hand they are more sensitive in the psyche, more open to impressions from the environment. It is also not uncommon for them to be more finely tuned in soul. 'Blue-eyed' has a connotation of innocence, openness, being without a hidden agenda and therefore also unprotected in situations that may not turn out to be good for them. Sensitivity towards sunlight at the physical level may thus also be seen as general sensitivity in the psyche.

Fair-skinned people, being thus sensitive and more easily impressed,

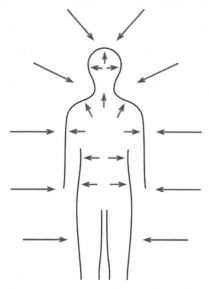

Form-giving powers from inside and impressions coming from outside act on the skin

need more inner protection. First of all they need the obvious protection from sunlight, but then also protection against too many impressions quite generally. Lack of this may increase the risk of melanoma.

This gives us something which people with many moles and those with fair hair and skin have in common – the need to protect themselves from the sun in particular and too many impressions in general. Without this, the risk of melanoma rises.

But how exactly does the connection arise between sun and melanoma, influences from our surroundings and melanoma?

In health, a balance is maintained in all body boundaries between the organism's own powers from the inner microcosm and forces coming from outside, from the macrocosm. The skin forms a boundary with that balance, which gives human beings their specific form.

At the level of the psyche, human beings live consciously in this interplay between inner and outer. They must actively seek to maintain a balance between being centred, inwardly focused, for instance in thinking of past experiences, and being out of themselves, for instance in listening to and taking in music. Imbalance arises when someone only allows things that are already known to him to count in a conversation, for instance, and does not listen to what the other person is really saying. On the other hand we are also out of harmony if we are nothing but open, taking in everything that comes to us with excessive sympathy.

This situation where influences from outside are predominant at the organic level often exists for melanoma patients. Forces coming centripetally towards the human organism grow too powerful and push back the organism's own powers of form. Foreign powers of form break in; sunlight is only a (greater or lesser) part of the broad spectrum of foreign elements. The process upsets the subtle interplay between matter and form in the human skin. Cancerous degeneration develops, a 'catastrophe of form'. The pole of matter is no longer controlled by the organism's form principles; cells multiply of their own accord, formlessly, and a tumour develops.

Once a dermatologist has seen a fairly large number of patients with melanoma, he will often find a specific type with particular mental traits.

Melanoma patients are subtle, sensitive, and perhaps thin-skinned. Their inner life tends to be rich. They're not for 'roughing it', for coping staunchly in any situation. One often finds them open to others. They have an open ear for the problems of colleagues, a heart for the problems of other nations. This may lead to increased social commitment, to the point where they take on too many voluntary positions.

An inherited skin disposition (fair skin type, many pigmented moles) and a particular type of character are often the conditions under which people are liable to develop melanomas. (There are also others who do not have any of those characteristics but do have melanoma.) Specific events in life will often make the melanoma manifest – stress at work or at home, strokes of destiny, worries may precede the condition. Sudden mental stress causes a shift in the relative presence of forces in the skin, and the disease develops. Characteristically this happens frequently in the middle years of life. Professionally one has reached a high point, the family and home have been established, and so on. This is the stage of life where the outside world makes the greatest demands on people.

As with any skin condition that persists for some time and proves more limiting, the individual concerned will above all ask: Why has this happened to me? What do I have to do with this disease? It is, of course, possible to speak of individual factors which contribute to the development of melanoma, as has also been done above. Yet the individual is usually unavoidably and inescapably exposed to them. You cannot escape an inherited disposition, for example. And a person's biography, with periods when challenges and demands come to a peak, also has its own laws, though the individual is generally not much aware of this. Instead we speak of 'destiny', or 'fate', i.e. events and also diseases coming upon a person in the outer pursuit of his life.

When someone tries to gain sufficient insight into events and circumstances in his life, he can get an inkling that no satisfying expla-

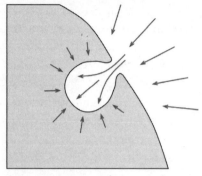

Form-giving powers from outside enter into the organism

nation for his destiny will be found if he considers only his present life. A biography must also have a history in the life which the soul knew before birth; the particular aspects of the present biography arise from that earlier life. In the same way, the evolution of existence in soul and spirit will not come to an end at death.

With melanoma, a serious illness, this means that the deeper reasons must always also be looked for in both the present biography and in a time that went before this. The thought of the human being continuing to exist after death suggests that the individual may well be preparing for future tasks in going through the disease. The destiny idea can be liberating and give courage to individuals who are looking for meaning. The horizon widens, coming free of the narrow confines of the present life. The individual who has the disease, his family and physicians and therapists must clearly do everything possible to cure the condition and change environmental factors that cause it. Once this has been done, however, we may also put our trust in the wisdom that determines our destiny.

The first measure in treating melanoma is surgery. The affected area must be excised with a good safety margin. The area has dropped out of the control of the organism's own form-giving powers; once it is removed, self-healing powers are able to come in more effectively. If the tumour is small enough to remove it under local anaesthetic, that is a definite advantage over full anaesthesia which is now known to weaken the immune system.

The immune system becomes intensively involved with the tumour. Mistletoe therapy can support this. Mistletoe is a plant with specific characteristics which give it powers to combat the tendency to tumour development in the human organism. Mistletoe products are manu-factured by a number of firms (Abnobaviscum by Abnoba, Helixor injectable solution, Iscador[1], Iscusin[2], and Isorel by Novipharm); they are injected subcutaneously or, less often, given by intravenous infu-sion. A physician with experience in mistletoe therapy will be able to decide which preparation should be used in which strength in a given case. It is recommended to start mistletoe therapy even before surgical removal.

Treatment with mistletoe preparations has been the heart of anthroposophical cancer treatment from the time when on the basis of his spiritual-scientific investigations Rudolf Steiner suggested its efficacy in treating cancer. Mistletoe extracts will not only enhance immune responses; they have constituents that can kill tumour cells or inhibit their growth. Special mention must be made of the distinct effect mistletoe has on patients' general condition, also evident to carers, and on the psyche. Mistletoe lifts depression, maintains a positive feeling for life, and helps to overcome the existential crisis which arises for anyone who suffers from cancer. It therefore helps in the process where the individual ultimately comes through the disease unscathed in soul and spirit, having matured in the process. We are therefore able to say that mistletoe is a medicinal plant with comprehensive actions against the tumour process. Ongoing research by the manufacturers is designed to improve pharmaceutical methods and hence the actions of their mistletoe products. Further information may be obtained from www.lukasklinik.ch.

At a cancer congress in Berlin in 2004, a trial with mistletoe therapy of malignant melanoma was reported. At 35 centres in Germany and Switzerland (mainly skin clinics and a few dermatological practices) 738 high-risk melanoma patients were compared; 381 had been treated with Iscador P (Weleda preparation of mistletoe from pine trees), 357 were not given mistletoe. Follow-up was for three years. The outcome of the trial clearly showed that preventive long-term treatment of melanoma with mistletoe after surgery reduces the risk of dying of melanoma and increases the chances of the melanoma not recurring.

In addition to mistletoe therapy, attempts may also be made to harmonize the interaction of powers of matter and powers of form by using potentized medicines. Antimony, Quartz and Formica may be considered (P).

Anthroposophical treatment of melanoma may also include eurythmy therapy. This is a movement therapy developed by Rudolf Steiner, the founder of anthroposophy, and based on the laws and creative powers of the human organism. It is a variant of eurythmy as a performing art. Instead of being directed outwards to an audience its actions are directed inwards for the individual who is doing the eurythmy therapy exercises. Movements of the body and limbs have healing potential extending to the sphere of internal organs. With melanoma patients, the aim of the exercises will be to stabilize the boundaries of body and soul and make them functional again. The powers of individual nature need to be strengthened in their actions at the organic level. The relationship to the outside world is gradually cultivated in the exercises so that it is taken up in a more conscious and balanced way. This helps to find the right middle position between being open and giving oneself up on the one hand, and closing oneself off and rejecting the world on the other.

Art therapy also comes in here. Painting therapy offers exercises in working with light and darkness, with penetrating radiance and the setting of limits, to strengthen powers of self-healing.

When someone with melanoma shows the character traits described above, one will advise him to endeavour to regain mastery over impressions coming from outside. The occurrences of modern every-day life, often hectic, must not overpower him. To use a maritime metaphor, the mountainous waves of events should not break over the individual human being; he must keep his head above water. How can this be done? The answer is that one must take care to 'digest' all the impressions received, work through them inwardly.

Ralph Waldo Emerson said that the heavens are the eye's daily bread, pointing out that impressions gained of the natural world feed us. In the words of Angelus Silesius, referring to the food that is our sustenance: 'Bread [alone] does not feed us; what feeds us in the bread is God's eternal word, is life and is spirit.' These words may also apply to the much more subtle sustenance we receive through the sense organs. In this sphere, too, 'life' and 'spirit' are behind the things we take in from outside. We need to release life and spirit from anything we take in through the eyes, for instance, and that needs inner activity for external light to become inner light, to give 'light' to the thinking human being.

This provides practical suggestions for everyday life. To master and stay on top of the multitude of impressions gained on a trip to Greece, for instance, it is a good idea to keep a diary, writing things down every evening, and to have a guide to Greek art and architecture to hand. If the impressions of ancient sites are not to be merely consumed, which ultimately leads to disease, one must be informed and educated on the subject. This enables one to appreciate the architectural idea of the Greek temple when visiting the ruins of antiquity, immersed as they are in the blinding light of the Mediterranean sun.

Inner activity thus makes it possible to oppose external light with inner light. This provides a kind of 'endogenous [the body's own] protection from light'. People with melanoma risk, or actual melanoma, must take care to avoid all stress in body and soul. They must find ways of thoroughly digesting all impressions coming from outside.

Protection from light is, of course, also needed on the outside. Preference should be given to protective clothing and a hat rather than high-factor sunscreen products. Those factors prevent sunburn from developing to warn us. As a result people stay in the sun longer, and parts of sunlight that are not filtered out, e.g. the UVA and infrared radiation, reach the skin in high doses. (It is not yet known what role these parts of light play in producing skin cancer.) It may also be the case that the chemical substances used for those sunscreen factors are taken in via the skin, and the metabolism then has to cope with foreign matter.

In the individual case, chemotherapy must be considered in consultation with one's dermatologist. The drawback of chemotherapy is that damage is not limited to tumour cells. The cytostatics (cell-destroying drugs) extend their anti-life action to the whole organism, also suppressing the body's own defences.

Another negative side to chemotherapy is that it inhibits life in soul and spirit. It makes it more difficult to gain the inner maturity which is won by coming to terms with the disease. This adds to its deep-seated causes. The effect of cytostatics on the psyche corresponds to their actions at organic level, for chemotherapy will often prove carcinogenic itself.

Information on the essentially standardized conventional treatment is widely available.

Basal cell carcinoma

Two kinds of skin cancer develop from the cells of the epidermis — basal and squamous cell carcinoma.

Basal cell carcinoma is the most common form of skin cancer; it does not produce metastases but can spread, ignoring organ boundaries, and go down deep if it persists for years or decades. Other forms of basal cell carcinoma may branch out through skin tissue and soon spread sideways. Dermatologists usually identify basal cell carcinoma by its characteristic appearance. The margin is raised, producing a pearly border; the lesion consists of small nodules covered with very fine blood vessels.

People with light-coloured skin sensitive to the sun are more likely to develop the condition. Chronic sun damage to the skin makes the body's own powers of form falter after decades, and the horn cells in the epidermis then develop shapeless bulges. The condition develops mainly in the sixth to eighth decade, affecting primarily the areas in the face that are exposed to light. It is less often found on the trunk.

Basal cell carcinoma should be removed under local anaesthesia as early as possible, when it is still small. The removed tissue is examined under the microscope, looking particularly at the margins of the lesion to make sure the whole of it has been removed. If the degenerated tissues do not stop short of the margin in the excised material, further surgery will be required. In people of great old age, for whom the operation would be too much, the tumours are treated with superficial irradiation. One may also try mistletoe therapy in such cases, injecting the preparation directly under the tumour (P). People who have had one basal cell carcinoma may easily develop another, generally in a different skin area and independent of the first. The possible need for preventative mistletoe therapy must therefore be considered in the individual case (P). If yes, it is given in courses, using series of injections in spring and autumn.

Squamous cell carcinoma and actinic keratosis

This form of cancer arises from the horn cells in the epidermis and initially tends to cornify. Like basal cell carcinoma it invades deeper tissues. Unlike basal cell carcinoma it may produce metastases in the relevant lymph nodes. This happens much less often and much more slowly, however, than it does with melanoma. Squamous cell carcinoma is promoted by sunlight. Affected age group, skin type and location are therefore the same as for basal cell carcinoma.

Squamous cell carcinoma often develops from a disorder of corni-fication (actinic keratosis) in ageing skin (see section on the ageing skin, pages 117–119). The lesions present as pink patches, usually less than half a centimetre in diameter, under a firmly attached cornified scale which may grow into a regular little horn. One quarter of these lesions degenerate into squamous cell carcinoma, which is why they must be kept under observation.

Squamous cell carcinoma must also be removed early. Mistletoe therapy may be used to treat metastasization or to prevent it (P), or to prevent further squamous cell carcinomas developing, much as in the case of basal cell carcinoma (P). Birch Cream (manuf. by Birken GmbH) is recommended for treating actinic keratosis, sun damage on the lips (usually the lower lip) and light-damaged skin quite generally. Apply over the whole area mornings and evenings (S). Betulin, the main active principle in birch cork extract, can promote the destruc-tion and removal of light-damaged horn cells in the epidermis.

Folliculitis (infection of hair follicles)

Hair follicles and their sebaceous glands are sites of intensive sub-stance creation. If this goes beyond a certain measure and the flow of substance to the skin surface – metaphorically speaking – gets too juicy, a tendency to get inflamed develops. This provides the right soil for bacteria, generally staphylococci, to invade the follicle and produce inflammation and pus. Pustules (with yellow heads) are seen, with a hair growing from them; the surrounding area is reddened. In men, the condition typically develops in the beard region and hairy scalp. It may, however, also appear anywhere on the body in both men and women.

The causes may be metabolic problems in diabetics; sluggish liver and/or intestinal function are other possible causes. In some people the pustules develop if they are using an ointment that is too greasy.

If the inflammation is fairly severe, homoeopathic preparations of bee (Apis mellifica) and deadly nightshade (*Atropa belladonna*) are recommended; use for a limited period – one or two weeks – as directed by your physician. If necessary, liver and intestine must be treated for a longer period to activate them (P). Externally, Calendula Essence$^{1/2}$ (lotion) in a zinc suspension (calamine lotion) has a soothing action (S).

Boils (furuncles)

A boil develops when folliculitis spreads to surrounding tissues. The painful, pea to hazelnut sized nodule is red, as are its surroundings. Within days, the centre melts down, the boil gets a yellow head, and pus is finally discharged to the outside. If boils appear repeatedly for years, in different parts of the body, the condition is called furunculosis. Diabetes encourages boils. In most cases, however, overweight is the real cause.

The fat in the subcutis gives the organism the potential for generating heat, as described in the first chapter (pages 14–15). No more heat should be generated, however, than the I, the spiritual level of human existence active in the organic sphere, is able to control. If too much fat has accumulated in the physical body and the spiritual governing principle is therefore no longer in control of heat generation, uncontrolled small heat foci develop, sites of inflammation, like small fires in the body periphery. This is how furunculosis may develop.

It is advisable to reduce weight when overweight and boils combine. Limit fat and protein (meat, cold meats, fish, eggs, dairy products). Pork in any form should be strictly avoided. To get the tendency to inflammation under control, red ant (Formica) may be applied externally, using high dilutions in a bath (P). In woodlands, it is the function of ants to take everything that is about to drop out of the regular cycle of vital functions to their ant heap and process it to maintain the cycle of live matter. In overweight people, Formica can bring fat that is independently following its tendency to produce inflammation back under the control of self-healing powers.

In the acute stage, it is again helpful to take Apis and Belladonna. Apis Belladonna or Apis/Belladonna cum Mercurio Globuli[2] are suitable for self-medication; 10 pilules to melt under the tongue every two hours (S). Snake venom may be needed (Lachesis), ideally injected subcutaneously (P). Externally, an ointment such as Ichtholan (manuf. by Ichthyol) can help bring the boil to a head and release the pus (S).

Heilsalbe Ointment[2] or Mercurialis comp. Ointment[2], which contains dog's mercury, have a similar action (S).

Boils on the face that are above the line from corner of the mouth to ear lobe must absolutely never be squeezed. There is a small vein in the upper part of the face that connects with major blood vessels in the brain. Bacteria can spread by this route and cause thrombosis.

Abscesses

When inflammation causes a more extensive melt-down of tissues in the dermis and sometimes also subcutis than with a boil, the condition is called an abscess. Staphylococci are the most common bacteria to play a role in this. Pus forms at the centre which must be discharged to the outside. A hot, red and painful swelling arises which may vary in size. Pulsation in time with the heartbeat may be present. Once the pus forms a central lake in the abscess, it is easily felt to be a fluid that can be pushed to and fro by finger pressure. Abscesses that develop around splinters are due to foreign-body reactions. They may also form around the body's own structures such as sweat glands, sebaceous glands or hair follicles. Areas most often affected are axils, the folds under female breasts, groin, genital region and gluteal fold.

With an abscess it is important to ensure the inflammation does not spread and that the pus can be discharged to the outside as soon as it has formed. If it does not break through to the outside by itself, the physician must open the way for it by making a small incision. Apart from this, all the products mentioned for treating boils can be used.

Epidermal cyst (wen, milia)

A cyst develops when surface skin gets into the dermis, due to an injury, for instance, or a hair follicle gets trapped. Sebum and cornified (milia) matter are then discharged to the inside rather than the outside, and the cyst will slowly grow. The contents are white and granular. A wen may develop on the face or trunk; the most common site, however, is the hairy scalp, where quite a number may sometimes appear. The cysts are pea to plum size, elastic to touch, with no sign of inflammation. On the scalp they may be a problem when combing one's hair. If a cyst should get inflamed it may develop into an abscess and discharge its whole contents in a self-healing process.

If a wen proves a bother it can easily be removed with a small incision made under local anaesthetic. The physician or surgeon will endeavour to remove every bit of the cyst, to prevent a new one developing.

Impetigo

Impetigo is seen mostly in children, especially in the warmer season. Often starting from a cold, streptococci, or more rarely staphylococci, infect the skin surface, causing red spots with honey-coloured crusts (bullae). The face is most often affected, but so may any part of the body, with the infection transferred by the hands.

The tendency to develop impetigo is above all seen in children with dry skin and a tendency to develop neurodermatitis. Earlier damage has weakened the skin's defences against germs. To a degree, however, impetigo may be infectious for any other child, which is why the condition sometimes occurs among several children in kindergarten or lower classes of primary school.

Pot marigold (*Calendula officinalis*) is particularly suitable for the external treatment of impetigo. Calendula has real healing powers, especially with purulent skin conditions. Use compresses with Calendula Essence[1/2] (1 tablespoon to $\frac{1}{2}$ litre of water) or Calendolon Ointment[1] (S). Antibiotic ointments are only rarely needed (P). Keep the affected areas really clean; Calendula Soap[1] is particularly good for washing. Internally, the physician may prescribe Apis and Belladonna; constitutional aspects that provide a soil for impetigo must be dealt with on an individual basis (P).

Erysipelas

This is an acute inflammatory process. Streptococci reach the dermis through some inconspicuous entry gate — perhaps a crack caused by fungal infection on the foot — and find a suitable soil in the ground substance between connective tissue cells. The affected area grows red, the patient develops a temperature and rigors, and the relevant lymph node grows enlarged. Erysipelas may recur, with the signs of inflammation less on each occasion. The persistent inflammation can then block the lymph vessels that drain the skin area in question. The consequence is a permanently swollen leg – a dreaded complication of recurrent erysipelas.

In most cases, anthroposophical physicians will not be able to deal with the situation without recourse to chemical antibacterial drugs. Bed rest is required. Externally, compresses with high-proof alcohol and chamomile tea give relief. The entry gate, e.g. the fungal infection on the foot, must also be treated. Internally, the physician will use Apis and Belladonna. If there is a tendency for the condition to recur, Quartz in homoeopathic preparation will call up powers of form in the dermis, so that the jelly-like ground substance will be under more effective control again (P). Externally, Brandessenz[2] (essence for burns) in quark (soft white cheese) applied directly to the hot, red skin areas, gives relief (S).

Being highly inflammatory and causing high temperatures, erysipelas was in the past used to treat certain forms of cancer. It was artificially induced by inoculation with streptococci, and in quite a few cases stimulation of the warmth organism and immune system led to improvement or even a cure of the cancer. Inflammation and sclerosis are polar opposites, and cancer counts among the cold, sclerosing diseases. The polarity explains the positive effect of erysipelas on tumours.

Another positive effect of erysipelas can be observed with leg ulcers (venous stasis). The open sore on the lower leg of someone with severe varicose vein disease, often persisting for months if not years, will quite often heal rapidly after erysipelas. The skin inflammation (erysipelas) causes increased blood flow to the area, and tissue growth can then start from the base of the wound and the sides.

Erysipelas thus quite often has effects which a physician who looks at things on a broader scale is able to appreciate.

Pityriasis lichenoides

The lesions appearing on the back, shoulders and neckline area are covered with small scales. After some weeks, if untreated also months, the colour changes from reddish to brownish to white. The reddish colour is due to mild inflammation, brown to the scales and white because the scales, gone by then, acted as a 'sunscreen' so that the underlying skin could not turn brown. A yeast called *Pityrosporum ovale* has multiplied greatly in the lesions (see also the section on Seborrhoeic dermatitis, pages 94–95). It exists in smaller numbers on normal skin, which is also why the condition is not infectious.

The cause lies entirely in the organism of the affected person, for this provides the nutrient basis the yeast likes. A disposition to seborrhoea (sebum flow with greasy skin) encourages the condition, and a physician will quite often find indications that liver function is sluggish. Pityriasis lichenoides is perfectly harmless, though it does tend to recur.

As a first step it is advisable to clear away the excessive yeast from the skin, for instance with Selsun 2.5% suspension (manuf. by Chattem). It contains sulphur and may be used like soap on the skin (S). In the meantime, liver function may be activated (P). Phosphorus in potentized form helps the organism to suppress the yeast of its own accord (P). After this, it will be best not to use skin care products with a high proportion of fat and avoid clothing made of synthetic fabrics that keeps out air. A preventive measure is a lotion containing Australian tea tree oil after showering (S). Sunlight in Australia has stimulated the tea tree to produce the oil and continues to be active in it. The yeast does not like it at all. Also effective are body washes to which rosemary has been added in the mornings and lavender at night; add a dash of the relevant Weleda or Wala bath lotion to the washing water (S). Silicea comp. colloidal Gel[2], which contains essential oil of lemon, and Birch Cream (manuf. by Birken GmbH) are also suitable (S).

Pityriasis rosea

The problem starts with an initially coin-sized 'herald' patch showing redness and scaling located on the trunk. A non-itchy skin eruption follows with oval red spots aligned along the skin tension lines. (Those lines mark the direction of main traction forces which act on the skin; the fine natural skin openings are also aligned along those lines.) The eruption is rather noticeable but quite harmless. It will resolve of its own accord in three to eight weeks.

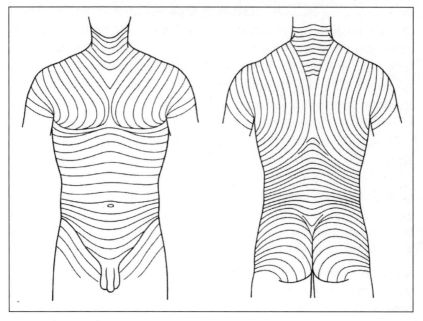

Tension lines in skin

The condition is more common in the winter season. The cause is not known. Infection has been suspected, possibly with a virus involving the skin, as with a childhood disease. Increased occurrence and fatigue with symptoms like those of a cold would suggest this. Stress also appears to play a role sometimes.

Pityriasis rosea can be irritated, which means that external treatment may make it worse. Body care products with a small amount of fat are recommended, or calamine lotion if the lesions itch (S). Dulcamara/ Lysimachia Drops[1], 10–20 drops three times daily before meals, can speed recovery (S).

Fungal skin infections – tinea corporis

Fungal skin infections are very common today. Up to a third of the Central European population have athlete's foot, up to a third of people over 40 have infected nails. Apart from the yeast *Pityrosporum ovale* (see page 134), which is normally found in low density on the skin, any fungus causes disease on the skin by provoking more or less severe defensive reactions. Yeasts, moulds and dermatophytes are specialized to grow on human or animal keratin (horn). The first two are less common and will not be considered in more detail. Fungal hyphae (threads) can be seen in scales under the microscope. It is also possible to identify the fungus by growing it in culture plates. It will grow like mould when the skin scales are put on agar. The species of fungus can be determined from the growth patterns.

Fungi from animal skin scales usually provoke extremely violent defence reactions on human skin. A typical example is that of a farmer who gets ringworm off his calves. A circular lesion with redness, swelling and scales develops on the trunk or arms and may even weep. The term ringworm comes from the slightly raised border of the lesion which is clearly defined, more red in the margin and spreads centrifugally. Children often catch the infection from cats and dogs. It is usually a genuine infection, for the fungus is very much present on scales from the animals, and the person who catches the infection needs no special disposition.

This is different when the groin is affected in an obese older person. The damp, moist environment in the groin then plays a role. Skin touches skin, sweat cannot evaporate, and the cornified layer of the epidermis softens. The fungus then finds ideal growing conditions in skin that is already partly damaged.

Diabetes also predisposes to fungal skin infection, in this case often with yeasts. The appearance is a bit different then, with a spread of small red nodules and spots around the reddened, often itching lesions.

No natural substance has so far proved completely effective in killing off dermatophytes on human skin. Antimycotics (synthetic products that kill fungi) must therefore be used if one wants to deal with the situation quickly. An antimycotic cream from the pharmacy is applied to affected areas once or twice daily (see directions on the package leaflet); the cream is prescribed by a physician. The action of antimycotics is rapid and effective.

Fungal skin infections – athlete's foot (tinea pedis)

Children rarely have athlete's foot. In adults the condition is getting more common following visits to swimming pools or saunas and/or due to wearing shoes and hosiery made of synthetic materials. Shoes and socks of synthetic material make the foot 'stew in its own juice' – which breaks down the cornified layer of the skin. The fungus flourishes in the darkness and damp warmth. The feet and sports shoes of professional footballers are a good example. Firmly tied shoes made of synthetic fabric and frequent training producing much sweat make the sports shoes into 'fungus containers' and ensure that more than half the players get infected. This has recently been shown as the result of a systematic study. In mild cases the fungus usually sits between the toes and will at most extend also to directly adjacent areas on the sole and the back of the foot. The cornified layer is often softened between the toes, with lamella-like scaling in the marginal areas and variable degrees of inflammatory reaction.

Here the causes are wholly external. It is different when large areas of the feet are affected. The soles of both feet and the sides are reddened and scaly; the toenails may also be involved. In this case there may be a particular inner disposition. The liver, its function to transform dead into live matter, may be sluggish. In the skin this causes problems at the surface, where live matter changes into dead in the cornified layer. When something is not properly enlivened from within, which means that the organism's own powers are not wholly present, microorganisms will unfold their foreign life.

For tinea pedis of moderate degree, the first choice for external application is Birch Cream natural (manuf. by Birken GmbH). The birch cork extract it contains can inhibit fungal growth (S). Another possibility of getting rid of the fungus without resorting to chemical drugs is Silicea comp. colloidal Gel[2], used in the mornings, with Cuprum metallicum prep. 0.4% Ointment[1] or Red Copper Ointment[2] thinly applied to the whole foot to above the ankles at night (S). In addition footbaths, as hot as possible, with Weleda or Wala Rosemary Bath Lotion added, three times a week (S). If this does not prove fully effective, you may have to fall back on one of the usual antimycotics.

If the infection has spread and the physician gets the impression that there is a disposition from within, he will look for the causes and if indicated treat the liver as well, for example (P). Gentian Stomach Tonic[2] would be suitable for self-medication, a teaspoonful three times daily for six weeks. It is helpful to avoid refined sugar and white flour. Phosphorus dissolved in oil and applied externally to the affected skin will change the foot environment, making it less favourable for the fungus (P). Phosphorus is a substance closely related to light. Reinfection is made more difficult. Foot Balm[1], Dr Hauschka Rosemary Foot Balm and Australian tea tree oil have similar preventative effects.

Measures to take with athlete's foot:
- wash feet every day; dry thoroughly, especially between the toes, using a hairdryer if necessary
- use fresh cotton or wool socks or stockings every day; wash these at a temperature no lower than 40°C
- never walk barefoot in swimming baths, wear bath shoes
- airy shoes of leather or other natural materials; change wet shoes
- do not wear shoes that are too tight; this reduces blood circulation and favours fungal infection
- disinfect shoes with Batrafen powder (ciclopirox olamine) once a week
- apply antifungal ointment for about eight weeks; when all signs of the infection have gone, continue to apply for two more weeks.

In summer it can happen that if there is fungal infection between the toes, or also without this, severe inflammation develops between the toes, partly due to bacteria, with redness, weeping and unpleasant odour. The skin comes away in thick lamellae in adjacent areas on the soles and back of the foot. This weeping inflammation improves quickly with footbaths using potassium permanganate and Tannolact (manuf. by Galderma) alternating daily, followed by application of Birch Cream natural (manuf. by Birken GmbH) (S). The betulin in the cream has distinct antibacterial action. Foot Balm[1] acts as a preventative (S).

Fungal infection of nails (onychomycosis)

Fungi and their hyphae (threads) can spread to the nails from the epidermis; this is most common in toenails, with the big toe usually affected first. The hyphae may be superficial, growing out from the outer end of the nail, or penetrate the whole nail plate and quickly reach the nail bed. The affected parts of the nail grow yellow, thickened and crumbly.

The condition develops where the enlivening, constructive and nourishing interplay of blood and nerve is disrupted, for instance if there are circulatory disorders (e.g. varicose veins) and nerve damage (e.g. in advanced diabetes). Damage to the nail itself through injury or constant pressure from (usually fashionable) shoes that are too tight also play a role.

The suggestions made for external treatment of fungal skin infections apply even more so for the nails. If you really want to be rid of the fungus, synthetic antimycotics will be needed (P). If the condition is only superficial, an antimycotic nail varnish will be sufficient (Batrafen, manuf. by Cassella Riedel, or Loceryl, manuf. by Roche). If the fungal growth goes deeper, the nail may be removed using a 40% urea ointment (Mycospor Nagelset manuf. by Bayer). It is recommended to collaborate with a podiatrist who will grind away the affected part of the nails, which opens the way for the urea ointment. If the whole nail or several nails are affected, perhaps even on both feet, lasting results will only be achieved with an antimycotic taken by mouth (P). Parallel to this, phytotherapy with marian or milk thistle (*Carduus marianus*) to treat the liver is advisable (P). The synthetic antimycotic has to be dealt with by the liver; taking it 'costs' the liver extra energy. This challenges an organ which – as described in the section on athlete's foot – may actually have been one of the causes, by being weak, of the fungal infection. It is therefore most important to continue the search for a natural treatment of this infection that will not put a strain on the liver. If toenails are only mildly affected (only some nails affected and only at the front), it is worthwhile trying Silicea comp. colloidal Gel[2] in the mornings, and combine this with Cuprum metallicum prep. 0.4% Ointment[1] or Red Copper Ointment[2] thinly applied over the whole foot, to above the ankle, at night (S). As already mentioned for the treatment of athlete's foot, footbaths with Rosemary Bath Lotion from Weleda or Wala, three times a week, are part of the treatment (S). Nicotine consumption must stop completely to improve the circulation to the limbs. Taking biotin (a kind of vitamin, from pharmacies) stimulates new nail growth (S).

In the past, the affected nail would be taken out, but this has disadvantages. The extraction causes additional damage to the nail system, with the disposition to fungal infection increasing. And even if the extraction is carefully done, this does not exclude the possibility of the fungus growing into the nail again.

Common warts (verrucae vulgares)

Warts are thickened lesions in the epidermis caused by a virus in the horn cells. Children with dry skin and a tendency to neurodermatitis are liable to have warts. Adults have far fewer warts, and then usually in connection with poor circulation in hands and feet caused by nicotine, for example, in smokers. Warts cannot really be called infectious. The viruses go to where they find the right soil on someone's skin; one only sees them where the soil is right, therefore. Putting it the other way round we may say that someone with a disposition for warts collects the viruses for this anywhere he finds them. Those viruses are universally present, so one does not have to wait to get infected.

Common warts on the hands are the typical nodules with a rough, cornified outer surface. On the soles of the feet, the nodules are pushed into the skin by the body weight. The discomfort felt is as if there were a pebble in one's shoe, and they are also known as plantar warts. Warts are perfectly benign and heal of their own accord after a longer or shorter period of time.

Children's warts respond well to herbal medicines used internally and externally – Thuja occidentalis D3 (3x) dil.[1] (arbor vitae) and Berberis Fructus D3 (3x) dil.[1] (fruit of barberry), 10 drops of each three times a day before meals (S). Clear the way first for external application by softening the cornified part of the wart. Use two products, on the principle of 'two is better than one' –

1 Duofilm (manuf. by Stiefel UK; nitrocellulose lacquer with salicylic and lactic acid); paint on the wart, leave to dry;
2 Guttaplast (manuf. by Beiersdorf; salicylic acid plaster); cut to size and place on the wart;
3 cover with sticky plaster;
4 remove plaster after one or two days and scrape off the softened wart with the back of a knife; repeat procedure if much cornified tissue still remains (S).

Salicylic and lactic acid will soften the cornified layer. When this has thinned down sufficiently, apply Polygonatum 5% Ointment[1] (solomon's seal). Apply thinly to the wart at bedtime, for several weeks (S). If more cornified tissue has developed in the meantime, repeat steps 1–4 of the above procedure.

It is advisable to let a physician look at the warts first, so that one doesn't get mixed up and treat corns instead, which would be to no avail. Using acids for some time, one will also finally get rid of the warts. Electrocautery (use of heat) is a more radical method and only possible with local anaesthesia.

Molluscum contagiosum

A specific type of virus causes mollusca contagiosa to develop. The lesions are the size of a grain of millet with a small, just visible opening at the centre where one can see the waxy or pearly core inside. The viruses which cause the lesion are in there. Mollusca contagiosa are seen almost only in children who may have large numbers of them spread over the trunk and the parts of arms and legs that are close to the body. Like common warts, they affect mostly children with dry skin and a disposition for neurodermatitis. These lesions are no more infectious than are common warts. It is the condition of the skin, the soil which the virus finds, which decides the issue. The lesions will heal on their own; their disappearance is often preceded by inflammatory redness, and sometimes pustules may develop.

To speed up recovery you may use herbal medicines, for example arbor vitae, Thuja Tincture[1] for external use, or Thuja Essence[2]

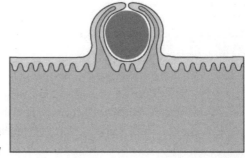

Molluscum contagiosum with horn body

dabbed on undiluted once a day and left to dry (S). Then apply a thin layer of Antimonite 0.4% Ointment[1] to the whole affected skin area (S). With older children able to control their fear of going to see the doctor, the small beads can be scraped out. It does not hurt, just a little nip. All mollusca contagiosa treated in this way heal up within a few days.

Condyloma acuminata

Condylomas are also caused by viruses and occur in moist, warm sites. They appear in the genital region and in the gluteal fold around the anus, and may also be found in the mucous membranes of the vagina and in the anal canal. Condylomas usually occur in fairly large numbers ranging in size from pinhead to bean-size or more. They are soft, and the shape resembles a fig or coxcomb.

Figwarts are passed from person to person on direct contact, usually during sexual intercourse. Their appearance indicates that the person's metabolism, especially in the pelvic region, is not adequately taken hold of by the higher levels of existence (soul and I).

For gentle treatment of condylomas you may try sitzbaths with Thuja Tincture[1] for external use and Polygonatum 5% Ointment[1] (S). Colchicum comp. Ointment[2] (with autumn crocus and greater celandine) is an alternative (S). In the past, a poison (podophyllin), heat or scraping were used, but these are not usually necessary nowadays, for it is now possible to stimulate the body's defences against the viruses. The synthetic drug imiquimod is used for this (in Aldara 5% Cream, manuf. by 3M Medica); it makes the affected skin cells recognizable for the immune system, which then breaks the cells down in a strong inflammatory reaction.

Herpes simplex

Herpes, usually on the lips, is also caused by viruses. A feeling of tightness, with itching or a slight burning sensation, is followed by a red spot, with a group of blisters (vesicles) developing on this. The blisters open and join up to form a weeping lesion with yellowy crusts. Redness will persist for some weeks as the lesion heals.

The first infection usually happens in early childhood, with the inflammation particularly violent as no specific defences against the virus will have developed. If the infection extends to the oral mucosa, painful open sores develop in the mouth and the condition is known as ulcerative stomatitis. The viruses lie dormant in the tissues for the rest of one's life and may appear again as the typical herpes blisters when provoked in various ways. The same skin sites are usually affected; apart from the lips, the condition may also affect the genitals.

Herpes may develop under the following conditions:
- febrile infections of the upper respiratory tract (fever blisters)
- when disgust is felt of something
- after intensive exposure to sun (glacial sunburn)
- in women during their periods
- with stress
- with an upset stomach, or nervous stomach
- following mechanical strain, e.g. dental treatment

Herpes can be made to heal more quickly with potentized medicines taken internally (e.g. Cantharis, a poisonous insect known as Spanish fly) or with herbal products applied externally (P). Extracts of lemon balm (Lomaherpan Cream manuf. by Lohmann) or of sage (Virus-Salvysat Solution, manuf. by Buerger) are suitable for external use (S). Both plants come from the mint family (Labiatae) and contain substances that can kill the viruses.

Some individuals get herpes blisters once a month or even more often. Homoeopathic medicines in fairly high potency can help to prevent this (P).

Shingles (herpes zoster)

Chickenpox is a typical childhood disease caused by viruses. When the infection with its typical vesicles in red spots erupting over the whole body, including mucous membranes, has died down, the virus is not completely eliminated. It lies dormant for years and decades in specific nerve cells in the spinal marrow, not causing any symptoms. When the organism's defences are reduced at some time, the virus gets active again, spreading from the spinal marrow to the nerves that ensure skin

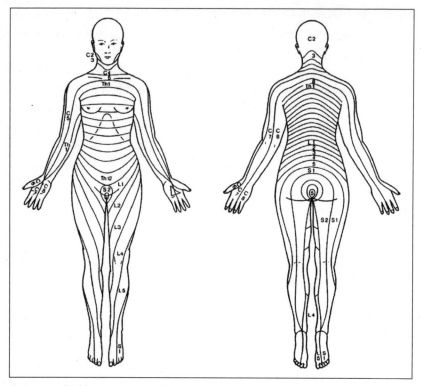

Areas supplied by cutaneous skin nerves (dermatomes)

sensitivity. The skin is then also affected, resulting in the typical shingles lesions – groups of vesicles on reddened skin areas. The condition gets its name from the way in which the skin changes are arranged in horizontal bands on the trunk, corresponding to the supply area of a skin nerve.

Shingles is a disease affecting two organic systems – a nerve and the skin area the nerve supplies. This explains the skin changes on the one hand and the neuralgic pain which often develops on the other. They disappear as the skin heals, but may also persist for months or even years, which is very hard for the individual in question. The sensory nerves of the head may also be affected. If shingles develops near an eye or ear, an eye specialist or ear, nose and throat specialist must check if the eye or ear is affected as well. If shingles occurs in a more widespread form (skin areas supplied by several nerve branches, single vesicles scattered over the whole body, or more deep-reaching skin damage underneath the vesicles), it is helpful to consult a specialist in internal medicine to exclude the possibility of something more serious (e.g. a tumour).

Mezereon (*Daphne mezereum*) in potency is the most important medicinal plant to treat shingles (P). Externally, a zinc suspension with Calendula Essence[1] dabbed on to the lesions is helpful (S). When crusts have formed, WCS Powder[1] promotes healing (S). Neuralgic pain is prevented or reduced with Aconite comp. Oil[2] applied to the whole affected area (S). Cover with a piece of cotton, which one uses again and again, so that it will gradually be soaked in the oil; use sticking plaster to hold it in place.

Scabies

The scabies mite is wholly 'specialized' in humans, living all its insect life cycles on human skin. It makes burrows up to a centimetre long in the epidermis, where it lives on the horn cells. The female mite is twice the size of the male; she is just about visible with the naked eye. To demonstrate that the mite is the cause of a skin eruption, a physician uses a fine needle to winkle out a mite; the mites are usually at the end of a burrow. The insides of the wrists, skin between the fingers, under the axils and in the genital region are most commonly infested. The mites are never found on the head or neck. The immune system needs four weeks to develop enough defensive powers to combat the mites, especially their faeces, and this results in a severely itching eczema. The itching gets worse in the warmth of one's bed.

Infection is always from person to person and needs intense bodily contact of the kind given with sexual intercourse, shared beds in the family home, or in nursing or geriatric care. The condition affects above all people with reduced defensive powers – children and old people, the sick, alcoholics. A healthy person with a good immune system exposed to numerous mites (e.g. a carer in an old people's home where the old people she looks after are seriously affected) will catch the infestation. Transmission is highly unlikely from just shaking hands or from the underwear and bedclothes of someone who is affected.

Lindane and permethrin are generally used in conventional dermatology to kill the mites. Both substances are also poisonous to humans, affecting above all the nervous system (lindane is by far the more toxic of the two). Neem extracts on the other hand are not toxic to humans; they come from the Indian neem tree and have been effective in fighting parasites for hundreds of years in India. Apply the neem extract as an ointment in the mornings, always after a bath. The 2% Neem Extract Ointment (manuf. by Trifolio M) is then applied three times a day as follows:

Day 1   head and extremities in the morning and evening, on the trunk at midday

Day 2   on the trunk in the morning and evening, on head and extremities at midday, and so on for a total of 10 days (S).

Underwear and bed linen should be boiled. Clothes that cannot be washed need to be aired for five days. The mites die when they have been away from human skin for three or four days.

Head lice

Head lice also live only on humans and are therefore always passed from person to person. As with scabies, lice infest mainly people whose defences are not yet fully matured or who are weakened. Head lice are a common problem in nurseries and schools. Infestation becomes evident because the bites itch, mostly behind the ears and on the back of the head; bites are lentil-sized reddened weals with a red dot at the centre.

Lindane is generally used or a pyrethrum extract (from chrysanthemums); both are also toxic for humans (lindane much more so). Lice are increasingly growing resistant to pyrethrum extract. Neem extract may also be used. Massage Neem Extract FT Shampoo (manuf. by Trifolio) into the damp hair and leave to act for 10 minutes. Do this three times in 10 days, on days 1, 3 and 10 (S). The extract inhibits chitin synthesis in lice (and also mites). Humans have no chitin metabolism, and so the extract is essentially non-toxic for them. The lice take in the poison as they feed. They do not die immediately but are unable to reproduce. This is why the treatment needs 10 days.

After using the shampoo, something must still be done against the nits; well-encapsulated louse eggs found sticking to the hair behind the ears in beige-coloured capsules just visible to the eye. The poison does not touch them. Remove the nits by repeatedly washing with tepid vinegar and water (1 part 6% vinegar in 2 parts of water) (S).

Dr Hauschka Neem Haarkur and Dr Hauschka Neem Hair Lotion are suitable for follow-up (S). Essential oils keep insects away; to prevent a new infestation it is recommended to massage a few drops of essential oil of cloves, rosemary, eucalyptus, geranium or lavender into the hair, in the case of children above all before they go to school.

To kill lice in clothes, cuddly toys, etc. the following alternatives may be used:

- wash for at least 10 minutes at over 60°C
- keep for 24 hours at a temperature below -15°C (freezer)
- keep in a plastic bag in a warm room for four weeks (the lice will have died of starvation then)

Insect bites and stings

Many different kinds of insects can irritate human skin as they suck blood or sting in self-defence. The sting or bite is followed by a swelling of lentil to palm size, with redness and a central red dot, the site of the actual skin injury. The swelling looks like the weals produced when we touch nettles. It is produced by the insect venom. It will almost always itch or burn.

An interesting observation is that it is always the same individual in a family, for instance, who gets bitten by insects, whatever kind of insect it may be. These individuals clearly have properties in the blood or give something off through their sweat or sebum glands which attracts insects. Others do not appear to have this attraction or at least much less of it.

Mites living on plants or in the pelt or plumage of animals are usually so small that we do not see them. They get on to human skin and bite in the search for nourishing fluids but discover that it is the 'wrong host' and depart again. All that is left is the itchy weal.

Trombiculiasis (straw itch mite infestation) is an example of mite infestation in August. Numerous tiny mites live on the vegetation in the natural world around harvesting time. They get on to the skin of people walking through woods and fields or doing harvest work on a farm and cause an itchy scatter of weals and scratched nodules. These occur mostly on the legs, sometimes especially in the region of the socks, with a clear limit set by the cuffs. They may also be on the abdomen, and in this case often limited by the line of the belt. A belt that fits closely stops them crawling upwards under the clothing.

The bites of horseflies and various other flies can cause skin infections, as the oral appendages of these creatures are often infected. Redness and swelling will then be more marked. The affected skin areas can also get very hot and lymph vessels going to the relevant lymph nodes may be inflamed. This can be seen as a red line from the bite towards the lymph node, which will be enlarged and painful on pressure. The popular term for this is 'blood poisoning'. Cooling compresses with Calendula Essence[1/2] (lotion, 1 or 2 teaspoons to $\frac{1}{2}$ litre of water) will prove helpful, as will immobilizing the affected limb. Medical advice should always be sought.

Ticks are not easily got rid off, and their bites may cause specific infectious diseases.

The insects sit among the grasses, on bushes and tree branches and drop down on to humans and animals when they perceive their odour. Their mouth parts are barbed. It is not advisable to use oil or adhesives, which are often recommended for removing the tick, for they may cause the creature's intestinal contents to get into the skin. Germs may get in that way. To remove a firmly attached tick, it is best to use forceps; take hold of the insect between its head and body, twist gently and withdraw. Pharmacies stock special tick-removing forceps that allow one to grasp the animal directly on the skin surface without squeezing its body.

Ticks may transmit microorganisms causing two different diseases. One virus causes tick-borne encephalitis (inflammation of the brain and its membranes); organisms called Borrelia cause Lyme disease. We will not go into detail about tick-borne encephalitis here.

Borrelia are closely related to the microorganisms that cause syphilis; 50 per cent of ticks carry the bacteria. In Europe, infection is to be expected only when the tick has been sucking blood for seven hours. Prevention is possible if you regularly examine yourself and members of the family after a walk, etc. in nature. If Borrelia are transmitted by ticks, the skin around the bite will be red, with the area clearly defined and growing week by week (erythema chronicum migrans = migrant redness). In the end, large parts of a limb or the trunk may be reddened. Spontaneous recovery happens at this stage. On the other hand the infection may cause degenerative inflammation in different organic systems (skin, joints, heart, liver, kidney, lung, brain). Antibiotics are therefore required; at the present time it would be too risky to try and deal with the situation by stimulating powers of self-healing only.

The numbers of people with allergic reactions to bee and wasp stings is growing. Being stung may for them cause a life-threatening allergic shock (instant allergic reaction) with hypotension, nausea, vomiting, dyspnoea (difficulty in breathing) and heart failure. People with and without an atopic constitution are affected with equal frequency. Anyone with a bee or wasp allergy should always have the necessary medicines to hand in case they are stung.

Desensitization is an effective treatment for allergy. Very small quantities of the venom are given by subcutaneous injection, gradually increasing the dose; these get the immune system used to the insect venom until finally a bee or wasp sting will no longer cause an allergic reaction. Anthroposophical medical constitutional treatment can reduce the organism's tendency to react to the venom with allergy (P).

The essential oils of clove, rosemary, eucalyptus, geranium or lavender help to prevent insect stings and bites of all kinds (S). Their scent takes away the insects' appetite, as it were. The itching from insect bites and stings is relieved using Combudoron Gel[1] or Wund- und Brandgel[2] (gel for wounds and burns) (S). If nothing else is available, Olbas Drops (a mixture of essential oils manuf. by Lane) or a silica gel will give relief if applied immediately (S). If the swelling is more severe, compresses with dilute Combudoron Lotion[1] or Urtica comp. Lotion[2] will have a cooling effect and reduce the inflammation (S). Internally, Apis/Belladonna cum Mercurio Globuli[2] may be taken, 5–10 pilules three times a day, to dissolve under the tongue (S).

Ingrowing toenail (onychocryptosis)

Frequently in younger years but also at any time in later life, the nail of the big toe may cause inflammation in the nail fold. The nail acts as a foreign body and the nail fold wants to reject it. Sweaty feet, cutting off

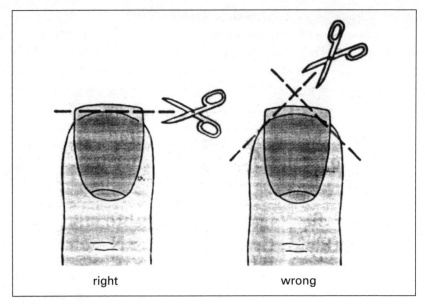

right   wrong

Cutting toenails

the outer corners of the nail and tight shoes, with moisture held in and pressure from the sides, will make the situation worse. Bacteria may also help to maintain it.

The nail must be cut straight across and not too low at the edge (projecting not more than 2 mm from the nail fold) or down the sides. It is also necessary to check if the skin has a particular tendency to get inflamed and treat this. Causes of this may be diabetes, overweight and a sluggish liver. Locally, use footbaths with potassium permanganate, tea tree oil on cotton wool and Heilsalbe Ointment[2], or Mercurialis 10% Ointment[1], applied in the thickness of the back of a knife and covered with a plaster (S). For the footbath, use a few crystals of potassium permanganate (from a pharmacy), which dissolve quickly on stirring; the water will be a brilliant violet in colour (S).

Recurrent aphthous stomatitis (mouth ulcers)

Chronic mouth ulcers that keep recurring are a common disorder; they are usually painful oval lesions in the oral mucosa (lining of the mouth) that tend to occur in groups. The causes have not been established in conventional medicine. Being closely connected with the moist, watery element, the oral mucosa evidently lacks powers of form and simply dissolves in those lesions. Potentized mercury (Mercurius) taken by mouth can stimulate those powers (P). Ratanhia Mouthwash[1] contains astringent extract of myrrh. Use a Q tip to apply in full concentration to the lesions. It will burn but just for a moment, and speed up the healing process (S). Another possibility is Echinacea comp. Essence Spray[2] (mouth and throat spray), a single spray action applied to the inflamed lesions several times a day (S). Liquid Mouth Balm[2] contains potentized antimonite; apply several times a day, using the pipette provided, or place cotton wool soaked in it on the site overnight (S). The method may be used to treat any kind of inflammation in the mouth and gums.

Yeast infection of the mouth produces a white coating, usually on the tongue. Suggestions for treatment are given in the section on Intertrigo. Brief mention may be made of mucocoeles (mucous retention cysts), a common condition. The lesion may be up to 1 cm in size, a blueish soft nodule full of fluid that feels elastic. It is most common close to the red part of the lower lip, and caused by the duct from a slime gland tearing due to mechanical stress. Mucus collects in the mucosal tissue. The lesion is quite harmless.

Changes may also occur in the tongue, a coated tongue being the most common. The oral cavity is the gateway to the gastrointestinal tract. Not surprising, therefore, that functional disorders of that tract leave their mark even there. Hairy tongue is an extreme form of coated tongue. The surface of the tongue is covered with a matted mass of papillae that have grown too long. Geographical tongue (benign migratory glossitis) is patchy and develops because cells desquamate (shed scales) at variable rates. A fissured tongue, not uncommon, merely has an unusual architecture. All the above are perfectly harmless in themselves, though they do give an indication to the expert of problems in the digestive tract.

Varicose veins (varices)

Arteries carry red blood, freshly charged with oxygen in the lung, from the heart to the periphery, to organs, muscles and the skin. Blue blood laden with carbon dioxide flows from the periphery back to the heart.

It has to go against gravity in the leg and pelvic veins before it reaches the large inferior vena cava and then the heart. At first this may seem miraculous, making us think that the blood must have its own dynamics. As in the rest of the organism, a struggle takes place especially in the blood between forces of gravity and buoyancy. In the human organism endowed with life and soul, the forces of buoyancy and of light must always have the upper hand. When this proves impossible, the external forces of physics prevail, and for the venous system this means stasis, with the blood too heavy and sluggish. This describes the beginning of a varix (varicose vein).

The following processes and organic structures support blood flow back to the heart. Contraction and relaxation of muscles in the legs and pelvic floor massage the veins, which makes the blood move. The rhythmical movement of the diaphragm creates negative pressure in the veins to move the blood towards the heart. The veins have valves that close like lock gates when blood threatens to move downwards under abdominal pressure when we laugh, sneeze, cough or pass stools. This prevents natural flow (to the heart) from reversing and taking a pathological direction (down into the legs).

How does weakness in the veins develop? Every second person in Central Europe has varicose veins to a greater or lesser degree, and these increase with age. Varicose veins are therefore 10 times more common among 70-year-olds than among people who are 30 or 40.

Family disposition plays a role. Constitutional connective tissue weakness leads to loss of elasticity in the walls of the vessels which then become enlarged. Not enough exercise, standing and sitting down for long periods helps to slow down blood flow in the legs. Tight-fitting clothing, tight jeans, for instance, and creases cutting into the flesh in the groin region when sitting act in the same direction. High-heeled shoes prevent the 'muscle pump' from working properly in the calves. Overweight adds to the forces of gravity in the body quite generally, with fat increasing the mass that exerts downward pressure.

The hormonal situation also plays a major role in the development of varices. They are twice as common in women as in men. Taking hormones to prevent conception (the pill) encourages the development of varices. Thrombosis is also more common on the pill, which in turn damages the veins and helps varices to develop. In pregnancy, the foetus presses on the veins in the lower pelvis, especially as much additional venous blood then flows around the uterus in pregnancy. Finally if the liver, one of the functions of which is to vitalize the blood, grows sluggish, this is another cause for the condition.

The symptoms which appear as blood flow in the leg veins slows down are pain and sensations of heaviness and tension in the legs. It is interesting to note that the severity of symptoms does not relate to the severity of the condition. A leg which looks quite normal from the outside may cause a lot of problems, and a leg with serpentine veins the thickness of a little finger none at all. The lower legs and especially the ankle region may swell up (oedema). Night-time cramp in the legs, pruritus and restless legs may torment the individual concerned. When varicose veins have persisted for decades, eczema may develop, with the skin showing brown discoloration and hardening in the lower leg, making the leg look like an upside-down champagne bottle. An ulcer may also develop in the lower leg.

It is never too soon and never too late to take preventive action if there is a tendency to varices. Excessive weight must be reduced. At work, alternate between standing and sitting down. It is good to do some walking in between, especially if emphasis is put on pushing the foot off the ground. Climbing stairs is very good for activating the muscle pump. Walking and cross-country skiing are good for prevention. Downhill skiing, jogging, hopping and weight-lifting aggravate the condition if there is a disposition. Kneipp treatments and treading water are helpful; mud or peat baths and exposure to the sun should be avoided. Eurythmy therapy encourages powers of buoyancy in the whole organism.

The most important principle in treating varicose veins is compression. Compression hose of adequate strength or — even better — compression bandaging may be used (P). To do the bandaging one needs two elastic bandages which are put on from foot to knee running counter to each other (e.g. Lohmann's Puetter Verband). Unna's paste or zinc gelatin bandage is particularly suitable with stasis dermatitis on the lower leg; the zinc oxide soothes the skin (P). Ready-made bandages are available from various firms.

Compression bandages must be put on first thing in the morning, as no oedema will have developed at the start of the day. Venadoron Leg Toner[1] or Skin Tone Lotion[1] applied to the whole leg is helpful for heavy legs (S). It contains arnica, an important medicinal plant in this case; do not use in cases of arnica allergy. An alternative is Dr Hauschka Rosemary Leg and Arm Toner (S). A bath with horse chestnut extract is also beneficial – Chestnut Toning Bath Soak[1], 2 or 3 tablespoons to a bath, not too hot, two or three times a week (S). Horse chestnut extract (*Aesculus hippocastanum*) may also be taken internally; it counteracts oedema and tones the veins (P). An extract of melilot (*Melilotus officinalis*) acts in a similar way (P). Borago comp. Globuli[2], 10 pilules to melt under the tongue three times a day (S).

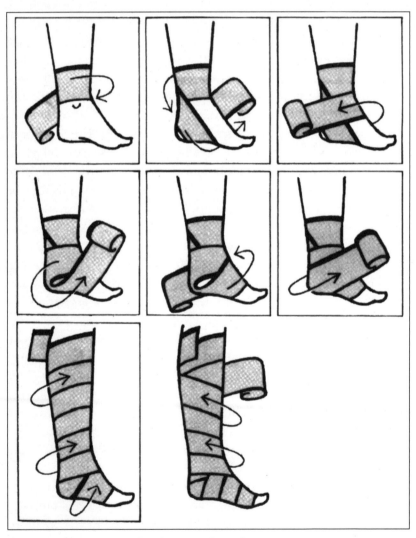

Technique of compression bandaging on lower leg

Once veins have become deformed, the physical damage cannot be made good without surgical or injection sclerotherapy. If surgery is used, the veins are removed and/or tied off; with injection sclerotherapy a chemical is injected that causes inflammation so that the walls become glued together. Neither method guarantees against new varicose veins developing in previously healthy parts of the venous system which forms a kind of net around the legs.

Complications arising with varicose veins

With superficial thrombophlebitis, the skin is reddened and hot, and a vein can be felt beneath which is painful and sensitive to pressure. Ointments containing arnica, compression bandages and physical movement are part of the treatment (P).

Deep venous thrombosis involves a slight rise in temperature. The leg swells up. In-patient treatment is needed in hospital because of the threat of pulmonary embolism if a thrombus (blood clot) from the inflamed vein reaches the lung. Postphlebitic syndrome may develop if the organism is not able to open the vein fully again after the thrombosis. Skin pigmentation then changes to brown, the skin hardens on the lower leg, and there is a tendency to develop dermatitis and leg ulcers (venous stasis ulcers).

With venous stasis ulcers, chronic stasis makes it so difficult to provide nutrients to the skin that the skin tissues break down. Treatment must be in the hands of a physician and is often prolonged.

Haemorrhoids (piles)

A third of the population have haemorrhoids, a common problem in our civilization. Haemorrhoids develop when the veins of the haemorrhoidal plexus in the rectum get enlarged. On the one hand, the rectum is closed by muscles forming a ring around the anus, like a fist keeping a sack closed. The result is closure which is strong but rather rough and ready. The venous plexuses under the mucous membrane at the very end of the rectum provide closure at a finer level, so that mucus and gases may also be retained. Too much blood in those veins enlarges them just as is the case with varicose veins in the legs. Soft nodules and pads develop, initially still inside the anus, but they may gradually protrude, first only after stools are passed and then permanently. If abdominal muscular pressure is exerted, as when passing stools, they fill up and are distinctly enlarged. The finer closure in the anus is lost, so that mucus may emerge. Pruritus (itching) and dermatitis may then develop in the gluteal fold. The haemorrhoidal nodules themselves may be painful (especially when passing stools) and discharge bright red blood (on the outside of the stools).

Poor intestinal motility and constipation are often found to exist together with haemorrhoids; the condition is made worse by a diet low in roughage and a largely sedentary lifestyle. The flow of blood from the small pelvis via the inferior portal vein back to the liver also tends to be sluggish, so that too much blood stays for too long in the venous plexuses of the lower abdomen. A sluggish liver may be contributing to the situation. The liver gets its name from 'to live'; it is the central organ in a living organism. It therefore also enlivens the blood and supports it in its own dynamics. A sluggish liver is like a weight resting on the blood, making it heavy. It is this heaviness of the blood which makes the walls of veins around the anus move apart.

Achillea comp. dil.[1] is made for dealing with this situation. Take 10–15 drops three times a day before meals (S). This medicine contains yarrow (*Achillea millefolium*), antimony, witch hazel (*Hamamelis virginiana*), horse chestnut bark (*Aesculus hippocastanum*) and yellow gentian (*Gentiana lutea*). Slow intestinal function and constipation can be dealt with by taking enough fluids and a diet rich in roughage, and eating biodynamically – or at least organically – grown produce. [In the UK, the wholesalers used by the supermarkets will label biodynamically grown produce 'organic'. Some 'organic' produce, esp. from Egypt, is quite likely to be biodynamic. Tr.] People who do sedentary work should make sure they get enough daily exercise. Ideally, stools should be passed at regular times each day. Symptoms are relieved with Haemorrhoidal Suppositories[1] or Quercus Haemorrhoidalzaepfchen[2] (haemorrhoidal suppositories) used after stools and before going to bed (S). Externally, Hamamelis/Stibium Ointment[1] or Quercus 5% Ointment[1] are a help (S).

More deep-reaching methods to change the physical situation are:

1   Injection sclerotherapy for early stages of internal haemorrhoids; the chemical is injected next to the haemorrhoid and the scar produced by the reaction will make the expanded vessel contract.
2   Rubber band ligation is used for larger internal haemorrhoids which protrude at stool; being tied off with the rubber band, the haemorrhoid dies.
3   Surgery is helpful in advanced cases.

Skin problems connected with pregnancy

The general condition and the skin bear the marks of the growth processes of the child in the uterus, for these radiate out to the whole maternal organism. It is not uncommon for a woman to feel better than ever during pregnancy. This outpouring of vitality over the whole maternal organism also involves increased water retention; the lower leg may be slightly swollen in the ankle region at night. Hair grows denser, longer and thicker, the nipples, genital area, groin and axils more brown due to increased activity of growing life. Fairly large hyperpigmented spots (melasmas) may appear on the forehead and temples; these disappear again (though not always) after the pregnancy. Varicose veins and haemorrhoids get more severe and can be a problem. This is partly due to mechanical causes – pressure from the growing foetus on the venous plexuses in the lower pelvis. On the other hand it may also be a sign that the mother's liver functions and forces of buoyancy in the blood are under stress, with gravity gaining the upper hand.

Stretch marks may develop in the regions where the maternal abdomen increases most in volume – on the stomach, over the hips and on the breasts. Connective tissue in the dermis, loosened by the extra water, opens up. Pre-existing skin conditions may improve or get worse during pregnancy.

• Adult acne will often heal; typical words of a pregnant woman: 'Never before has my skin been so beautiful.'
• With neurodermatitis, aggravations are in a ratio of 2 : 1 to improvement.

- The opposite is the case with psoriasis. Here improvement comes twice as often as aggravation.

A number of skin conditions are typical and specific for pregnancy. They may involve weals, vesicles, itching nodules, pustules next to small hairs, or just pruritus with no visible changes in the skin.

Skin changes of a more inflammatory kind, perhaps even weeping, will often improve if Dulcamara/Lysimachia Drops[1] are taken, 20 drops three times daily before meals (S). Antimonite D6 trit.[1] may be taken in addition, a good pinch three times daily before meals (S). These two medicines reduce the vitality of the blood in the skin. Pustules with yellow heads indicate the need to stimulate the liver. Take Fragaria/Vitis comp. Tablets[1], 1 tablet three times a day before meals and 2 at night-time (S). A percentage of pregnant women develop pruritus (itching) all over the body, usually due to bile blocking the small, thin bile ducts in the liver. Apart from taking Fragaria/Vitis comp. Tablets[1] in the above dosage, it helps to take Choleodoron Dil.[1] as well to stimulate the flow of bile, 10–20 drops three times a day before meals (if appetite needs to be stimulated) or after meals (if the appetite is too big already). The pruritus can be reduced by external application of Combudoron Gel[1] or Wund- und Brandgel[2] (gel for treatment of wounds and burns).

Skin conditions with diabetes

Metabolic diseases can also affect the skin. To illustrate this, we will consider diabetes and the skin conditions connected with it. Diabetes develops when sugar metabolism grows abnormal and too much sugar accumulates in the blood and is eliminated via the kidneys. The human I or self uses sugar to be wide awake and quick-thinking in the brain and to take action as needed in the muscles, which makes it the regent of sugar metabolism. Here it has lost control. Raised sugar levels damage the heart and all arterial blood vessels, including those in the eyes. Damage is also done to the metabolism in the nervous system and in the skin.

Too much sugar in the skin means a denser flora; think of a meadow given too much fertilizer so that some plant species produce a lot of green growth. The skin is too alive, and this leads to bacterial and fungal infection. Diabetics therefore tend to develop boils, with the inflammation a sign of excessive vitality. Yeast infections in the oral cavity, genital region, groins, gluteal fold and axils are also encouraged if the skin has too much vitality. The soil created for the yeasts is living sugar that is no longer under the full control of the human I.

First the diabetes must be treated, being the cause of the skin problem. Rosemary is used both internally and externally for this (P). Hot rosemary baths, also using the Junge Oil Dispersion apparatus, help the human I to establish a better connection again with sugar metabolism. Qualities of light and heat to which rosemary is much exposed in its natural Mediterranean habitat are taken into the plant and give it an affinity to the human I which lives in warmth. It then also does not come as a surprise to find that in the laboratory essential oil of rosemary also shows a slight but definite antifungal action.

The feet of diabetics are at particular risk when damage to nerves (polyneuropathy) and blood vessels (poor arterial circulation) combine. Both are caused by diabetes. Ulcers may develop, especially under the forefoot due to pressure. It is also possible for poor arterial blood supply to cause a whole toe to die off.

The following prevent complications in the feet of diabetics when these are at risk.

- Washing feet daily in lukewarm water (never hot, as loss of sensitivity means danger of scalding); footbaths with Dr Hauschka Sage Bath.
- Dry feet carefully.
- Apply Skin Tone Lotion[1] or Echinacea/Viscum comp. Gelatum (gel)[2] (both oil free) to the whole leg; if products containing oil are preferred, Rosemary 10% Ointment[1] or Rosemary 10% Oil[2] is recommended.
- Do not use external applications that irritate the skin.
- Check daily for injuries and fungal infection.
- Careful nail care using a file; never cut into the nail at the side.
- Inform your professional podiatrist of the diabetes.
- Wear shoes of soft leather leaving much room for play for the toes but a good fit at the heel and arch.
- Do not use tobacco in any form, as this narrows the blood vessels.
- Wear warm, wide socks.

External injuries

Skin injuries due to external factors (pressure, impact, cuts, punctures, bites, heat and acid burns) are not skin diseases as such. Many valuable suggestions are, however, available for home use and self-medication using anthroposophical medicines. Brief descriptions are therefore given of measures to take with external injuries. (All suggestions in this section are suitable for self-medication, the (S) marker is therefore omitted.)

Abrasions

Abrasions occur when an object with a rough surface strikes the body surface tangentially with some force, removing the epidermis and upper dermis. This opens the papillae of the upper dermis and their fine blood vessels (capillaries), resulting in the small droplets of blood typical of abrasions.

If the object which caused the abrasion was dirty (e.g. with a fall in a school playground covered with slag) the first step is to clean the wound. Use warm water and hard soap (curd soap); if necessary immerse the wound in the warm water to soften it a little before soapy water and a clean face cloth or soft brush are used to remove all dirt. This is most important, for particles of dirt may have got into the upper dermis where they may otherwise remain permanently. 'Dirt tattooing' may remain for life; it does not look good and must be prevented. Many of us have a small grey spot on a knee, reminding us of that painful fall in the playground years ago.

Compared to this, disinfecting the abrasion is less important. It is good to realize that the skin exists to cope with external insults; keeping out bacteria and making wounds heal are its natural functions. Disinfection is therefore only necessary with abrasions where a great deal of dirt has got in. For this, bathe in or use a compress with chamomile tea after using the soap and water. Pour $\frac{1}{2}$ litre of boiling water on two tablespoons of chamomile flowers, leave to draw for 20 minutes and allow to cool. If larger amounts of chamomile water are needed, it is better to use a commercial chamomile extract (e.g. Kamillosan, from pharmacies), diluting it according to manufacturer's directions. Chamomile (*Chamomilla recutita*) is a medicinal plant which apart from its healing action on skin and mucous membranes also disinfects. The use of products containing antibiotics or disinfectants is not advisable unless there is inflammation due to bacteria; both slow down wound healing. An antibiotic (from the Latin for 'against life') acts not only against bacterial life but also the life in the injured tissues. Chamomile on the other hand is a living plant the action of which is against bacteria only.

Having cleaned the wound, apply one of the following.

- WCS Powder[1] to dry the wound without plaster if there is no appreciable weeping or bleeding (do not use if hypersensitive to arnica);
- Heilsalbe Ointment[2] with or without a plaster; if allergic to balm of Peru, use
- Calendolon Ointment[1], Mercurialis 10% Ointment[1] or Mercurialis comp. Ointment[2]. These ointments are particularly suitable if wound healing is delayed and there is a tendency to suppurate. Pot Marigold (*Calendula officinalis*) is the most important medicinal plant for problems with wound healing and infected wounds; it stimulates healing from the base of the wound and initiates defensive processes. Dog's mercury (*Mercurialis perennis*) also deals with suppuration that goes deeper down, and may thus also be used to treat boils and abscesses.
- Calendula Essence[1/2] is helpful in compresses if the abrasion is followed by an inflammatory reaction from the organism and cooling helps. Use 1 or 2 teaspoons of the essence to $\frac{1}{4}$ litre of water.
- If a fat-free gel is preferred use Wund- und Brandgel[2] (gel for treating wounds and burns), but not if there is hypersensitivity to arnica.

Lacerations

Lacerations occur when the mechanical impact on the skin has caused a tear extending to the lower dermis or subcutis. A physician should always be consulted if the wound bleeds a great deal and needs a stitch or tissue adhesive to get good cosmetic results, especially if the wound is in the face. It is also helpful to consult a physician for lacerations on the hands, for many tendons and blood vessels are immediately beneath the skin in that area, and the injury may lead to complications. Lacerations over joints can also result in lasting limitation of mobility if scars cause the skin to contract. Otherwise lacerations are taken care of just like abrasions.

Cuts, puncture wounds and bites

Wounds caused by bites, punctures or cuts can go deep. The wound cavity is not open and germs are deprived of oxygen. This provides conditions for the growth of a particular kind of bacteria known as Clostridia. (These play a role in making silage in agriculture, when grass is fermented under exclusion of air. The organisms increase massively under those conditions, are present everywhere in the housing of silage-fed cows and also in milk. Hard cheese made from such milk will form cracks and break down, as the Clostridia produce gases.) The germ which causes tetanus is *Clostridium tetani*. The danger of getting tetanus thus exists particularly with cuts, puncture wounds and bites. Immunization against tetanus is therefore most important. It is comparatively less important with lacerations (though it should not be neglected) and least important with abrasions. If one wants to know if antitetanus protection is still effective following an earlier immunization, blood may be taken to have the antibody titre (blood levels of defensive proteins) determined in a laboratory. Protection usually is for much longer than was assumed until now, definitely more than ten years. Apart from this, cuts, puncture wounds and bites are taken care of in the same way as abrasions. The wound should always be allowed to bleed out as much as possible before treatment.

Once the open wound has healed, it is advisable to use Keloid Gel[2] to prevent excessive scar formation or hard scars. Apply twice daily, massaging the gel into the skin area until dry. The use of the gel is also advisable after operations.

Bumps and bruises

Bruises arise from blunt trauma. The skin remains outwardly intact; pressure causes blood vessels in the lower dermis and/or in the fatty tissues in the subcutis to tear, resulting in a bruise. This can be prevented from spreading by placing cold metal on the site (a coin, spoon, etc.). The coldness causes reflex contraction of the blood vessels; it also reduces the pain. Arnica (*Arnica montana*) is then applied. This is the most important and effective Central European medicinal plant for blunt trauma, and also for contusions, twists, sprains and even bone fractures. Before using arnica, it must, however, be established if the individual concerned is allergic to it, in which case it cannot be used. It should be added, by the way, that the allergic reactions to arnica seen in some individuals should never be the reason for banning the use of this plant for treating wounds externally in all people. The medicinal actions of arnica are so important that it must not be excluded. One merely has to know that allergic reactions exist and avoid using arnica with someone who has had such reactions, or stop using it if reddening and itching of the skin indicate that such a reaction is developing.

In practical terms, treatment with arnica may be in three stages:
- Measures taken in primary care for blunt trauma always must also relieve pain and reduce swelling. Apply compresses with dilute Arnica Essence[1/2], 1 tablespoon of the essence to $\frac{1}{4}$ litre of water.
- At the second stage, when the acute pain is less, change to Arnica Gel[1]; this maintains the cooling effect at a moderate level. Wala produce Arnica Wundtuch (wet wipes) which may be placed directly on the affected site. Both the gel and the wipes are useful for taking on rambles and journeys.
- When cooling is no longer required, or if it was not needed from the beginning, the use of Arnica Ointment[1/2] is recommended. The in-depth action of arnica can be assisted by putting on a dressing, possibly a piece of woollen fabric.

To get an idea of the medicinal action of arnica, consider that violence from outside upsets the healthy interaction of living body, soul and spirit in the human organism. The I, driven from the affected site to some extent, needs help from the powers of soul active in the body so that it may find its way back again. Arnica is the plant which can call on that soul activity which will enable the I to integrate again.

If arnica cannot be tolerated, it is recommended to use Cuprum/ Quartz comp. Ointment[2]. Apply twice daily and cover with a dressing. The ointment stains, so be careful of clothing. Here a combination of copper, quartz and essential oil of rosemary (*Rosmarinus officinalis*) does what arnica has been shown to do above.

To support the external use of arnica and help the bruising to disperse, Arnica, Planta tota D3–D61 drops may be taken, 5–10 drops three to six times a day before meals. The drops contain alcohol. An alternative is Arnica, Planta tota Rh[1], a solution in water available at the same potencies (D3–D6), or Arnica e planta tota D3–D6 Globuli[2], 5–10 pilules to be taken three to six times a day before meals.

Burns, scalds

With first-degree burns, the heat has only damaged the epidermis; redness and swelling develop. Healing includes a stage when scales are shed. If the whole epidermis is raised in blisters, which can be very large, we have a second-degree burn. The heat has also damaged the upper dermis, which secretes tissue fluid so that the epidermis is raised. No scars will be left. Third-degree burns cause serious damage to dermis, hair and nails. Hairs can be pulled out without causing pain, and pin pricks are not felt. Scars will remain.

Burns are treated in three stages:
- The first measure is to hold the burned skin area under running cold water; then apply a gauze compress or cotton cloth soaked in dilute Combudoron Lotion[1] or Urtica comp. Essence[2] (both are diluted 1 : 10 with water). Keep the compress moist by adding drops of the diluted medicament; if pain is severe, put ice cubes in the dilute solution.
- When the acute symptoms are less severe, a change may be made to Combudoron Gel[1] or Wund- und Brandgel[2] (gel for wounds and burns). Apply the gels thinly to the affected areas, repeatedly, and leave to dry.
- When a new epidermis has developed and the burnt skin is flaking off, treatment with Combudoron Ointment[1] may continue until the skin has fully healed.

Check for hypersensitivity to arnica before using any of the above products to treat burns. If the allergic tendency is there, Birch Cream (manuf. by Birken GmbH) is an alternative. Any blisters that have formed should be opened only if they are in an awkward site. It is advisable in that case just to pierce the blister and let the secretion run off through the small hole thus made. Left largely intact, the blister skin provides natural protection.

Sunburn

Sunburnt skin is red and swollen. Blisters may also develop. The fullness and power of sunlight (esp. the UV part of it) have caused a skin inflammation. The skin is burning, feels tense and painful, making it difficult to sleep at night. Rigors and a temperature may also develop.

Essentially sunburn is treated just like a burn:
- The symptoms of acutely reddened skin are most quickly relieved using compresses with dilute Combudoron Lotion[1] or Urtica comp. Essence[2] (both diluted 1 : 10 with water).
- When symptoms are less acute or if you are away from home, Combudoron Gel[1] or Wund- und Brandgel[2] are recommended. Apply thinly on repeated occasions and let dry.
- For follow-up treatment when the skin sheds scales use Combudoron Ointment[1]; this also relieves the itching which can be unpleasant.

Sunburn should be a warning sign that the individual has exposed his skin too much to the sun. It should never get as far as sunburn, especially in children, as the danger of developing skin cancer increases in step with the number of sunburns. The condition also reduces the defences in the whole organism and not only the skin. For prevention, wear textiles to protect from light – airy clothing and a sun hat. For areas exposed to light, Weleda and Wala both offer products made with mineral substances to protect from light. Metal salts (titanium dioxide and zinc oxide) are finely dispersed in a cream or milk and act like a sunshade for the skin. Compared to chemical factors, the metals are not taken up into the skin. The two Weleda products also contain an extract of edelweiss. A constituent of the extract captures 'radicals', substances which the alpine edelweiss creates to protect it from intense solar radiation. In the human epidermis, they capture the harmful chemical compounds formed on exposure to sunlight that encourage skin cancer.

Chemical burns

Strong acids or alkalis can cause chemical burns on the skin. Acids make protein coagulate and go solid; alkalis liquefy it. Acids are quickly neutralized, which stops their action. Alkalis penetrate more quickly and deeply into the skin because they liquefy tissues. They are therefore more dangerous (e.g. lime wash used on the walls of animal houses on farms).

The first step is to wash the skin area thoroughly under running water to remove the chemical. Any last residues and the secretions from the reactive skin inflammation are taken up by WCS Powder[1]. The powder, developed by anthroposophical physician Werner Christian Simonis, combines three members of the daisy family — arnica, marigold and *Echinacea* (*purpurea* and *angustifolia*) with quartz and antimony, which gives it excellent healing qualities.

IN CONCLUSION

Where internal medicine is concerned with diseases of the internal organs in the human organism, dermatology is concerned with diseases of the external organ, the skin. The fact that the skin lies on the surface of the body does not, however, mean that dermatologists treat only that surface. That would mean a danger of being literally superficial in their treatment. The author hopes that with the possibilities of treating skin conditions holistically which are discussed in this book he has contributed to removing that danger.

He has drawn on the wisdom of the anthroposophical view of the human being. This offers spiritual-scientific insights to help the healer and also the patient to look not only on the surface but more deeply at the human being in sickness and health. This opens up the view for the essential nature of the human being at the different levels of existence. We consider the world which is immediately apparent to the senses — the human body, the composition of its skin, processes in healthy and diseased skin — and recognize the spiritual which is at work in them. This alone makes it possible to understand and treat skin conditions in such a way that a higher state of health is achieved once they have healed. The special characteristics of the skin and deeper understanding of skin diseases also enable us to see our own body as a reflection of our individual nature with its own destiny. This is one way of gaining self-knowledge. The author hopes that readers will be able to see how illnesses, and especially conditions affecting the skin, offer an opportunity to gain in soul and spirit and to mature as human beings.

USEFUL ADDRESSES

United Kingdom
Anthroposophical Medical Association, Medical Section Office, c/o St Luke's Medical Centre, 53 Cainscross Road, Stroud, Glos GL5 4EX.
For information on anthroposophical medical practices, clinics and hospitals.

Birkencreme
Birken GmbH, Streiflingsweg 11, D-75223 Niefern-Oeschelbronn.
info@imlan.com
Details of products and how to obtain them, also in English.

Dr Hauschka Skin Care
Elysia Natural Skin Care, 27 Stockwood Park, Stockwood, Redditch, Worcestershire, B96 6SX. www.drhauschka.co.uk.
Very informative catalogue, list of outlets

Wala and Weleda products
Weleda (UK) Ltd, Heanor Road, Ilkeston, Derbyshire DE7 8DR.
www.weleda.co.uk
Information, catalogue, products.

USA
Physicians Association for Anthroposophical Medicine
1923 Geddes Avenue, Ann Arbor, MI 48104-1797. www.paam.net

Dr. Hauschka Skin Care, Inc.
59 North Street, Hatfield, MA 01038. www.drhauschka.com

Weleda
1 Closter Road, P.O. Box 675, Palisades, NY 10964. www.usa.weleda.com

Other countries
Internet search for any of the above should yield addresses in your part of the world.

FURTHER READING

An Introduction to Anthroposophic Medicine, Victor Bott, Sussex 2004
Medicine, An Introductory Reader, Rudolf Steiner, Sussex 2003

INDEX